The
Calcium
Factor

Robert R. Barefoot
Carl J. Reich

Book Reviews

"As a result of reading **The Calcium Factor** *I received excellent treatment and eventually cured myself of prostate cancer. I strongly endorse Mr. Barefoot as one of the top people in his area having excellent knowledge of nutritional therapy. I have yet to find anyone who has written such well-reasoned and scientifically based material,"* David G McLean, Chairman of the Board, Canadian National Railways.*"*

"In October 1996 I was diagnosed with prostate cancer. The diagnosis was confirmed by biopsy. In October of that year I started following Robert Bare foot's calcium regime. In July 1997 I had another prostate biopsy in which no evidence of malignancy was found. The regime outlined in the book **The Calcium Factor** *improves the immune system to where the body can heal itself, without intrusive measures like surgery, chemotherapy or radiation,"* S. Ross Johnson, Retired President of Prudential Insurance Company of America.

"I am a physician, with extensive credentials and honors that reach the White House and Heads of States in other countries. Mr. Robert Barefoot has worked over the past 20 years with many medical doctors The information has been culminated in two books, **'The Calcium Factor'** *and* **'Death by Diet'** *which have been used technically as Bibles of Nutrition. Mr. Barefoot is an amazing and extraordinary man who is on a 'Great Mission' for all mankind. I thank God for Robert Barefoot "*, Liska M. Cooper, M.D..

"Robert Barefoot's knowledge of calcium and it's alkalizing properties has been hungrily received by 100,000's of people throughout the world who are crying out to regain their lost health and vitality. Through his book **The Calcium Factor** *he has reached out to the common man in a language he can understand,"* Jill M. Wood, President Idaho Breast Implant Information Group.

Internet Reviews

"The most important Health book I have ever read".
(philratte@webtv.net, Minneapolis, Minnesota, May 19, 1999).
"This book proves how important it is to have the body fluids slightly alkaline and tells you how to test yourself so you maintain proper balance. It also proves that calcium is the most important nutrient after oxygen and water. Over 200 diseases, cancer heart disease, diabetes, etc., are linked to Ionic Calcium Deficiency. Calcium deficiency is the universal property of all cancer cells. Moreover, the production of mutation receptors cannot occur with the pH of the cell at the healthy, calcium buffered pH of 7.4.

"A Must Reading for those who lack calcium in their diet".
(oli@omninfotech.com, May 30, 1999).
"I was born a 'Jelly Baby' and did not walk until I was four years old. All through the years I have searched for the source of Calcium that works for my body. Mr. Barefoot certainly opened my eyes on the simple reality of a healthy body. He educated me on the most beneficial kind of calcium and how it is effectively absorbed in the body. Interestingly, he further introduced me to a simple technique in finding out the level of my health. I cannot tolerate lactose and the kind of Calcium he described in his book which I am now using is 'Heaven Sent'. Thank you!"

"Turned My Life Around". (Russell Vandorn, russell@newonthe net.com, California, October 12, 1999).
"I have been taking supplements for 20 years and engaged in athletic activities and working out. All was fine until a few years ago my body took a dive for no apparent reason. I tried lots of solutions with some help. Thirty days ago I read the book **The Calcium Factor** and then as instructed, acquired supplements. Like magic, the brown spots faded, my yellowing skin vanished, I lost excess weight, I regained new strength, my hair stopped falling out in the shower, I no longer get winded during exercise, and my eyesight is improving. I am amazed at what a dramatic effect the

right calcium formulation has had on me. I really feel as if I'm growing younger. My friends notice it too. If you do not at least read this book, which explains everything in qualifiable scientific detail, at least take supplements, the new age antidote to aging.

"Spellbinding Information". (nanjean, California, Dec. 13, 1999).
*"I could not put this book down. In **The Calcium Factor**, Robert Barefoot everything so clearly and everyone can understand this very important information. I want to scream 'WHY don't more doctors know this or pass this on !'. The research was done over 60 years ago and the medical profession continues to only burn, cut or poison (radiation, surgery, chemotherapy/drugs) the symptoms of disease like it was designed to do. As th back cover of the book states, 'cancer cells cannot exist in an alkaline environment', so if we put the body back into an alkaline state as it was when we were born, the cancer cells simple die off. Pass this book on to EVERONE you know."*

"The greatest preventive medicine book and real eye opener !". (betcruse@webtv.net, Bay City Oregon, November 9, 1999).
*"I cannot extol this book enough ! I have learned more in this little 138 page paperback called **Death By Diet** than I have in ALL the books, pamphlets, brochures, etc. that I have ever read. The knowledge, info and formulas for taking charge and gaining control of your own body's health and preventing disease is priceless! Makes complete sense. R Barefoot does an excellent job in explaining the technical parts of this book (remember, he is a chemist). My next book will be **The Calcium Factor** (same author). "*

"A very important, excellent book on health" (philratte@webtv. net, Minneapolis, Minnesota, May 19, 1999).
*"When I first read this book, **Death by Diet**, I was a little skeptical about some of the ideas presented. But now that I have used some of these ideas myself, I am most impressed with their importance for my health. I have also read his new book, **The Calcium Factor**, and it is even better. I love these books."*

iv

THE CALCIUM FACTOR:

THE SCIENTIFIC SECRET OF HEALTH AND YOUTH

BY

ROBERT R. BAREFOOT

AND

CARL J. REICH, M.D.

The Calcium Factor
The Relationship Between Nutrient Deficiency and Disease
By
Robert R. Barefoot & Carl J. Reich

Published By:
Triad Marketing
PO Box 590
Southeastern, PA 19399-0590

Copyright © 2000 by Robert R. Barefoot,
First Printing November 1992, Second Revised Printing August 1996, Third Revised Printing April 1998, Fourth Printing August 1999. Fifth Printing December 2000. Printed in Canada

Library of Congress Cataloging in Publication Data
Barefoot, Robert R.
The Calcium factor, The Relationship Between Nutrient Deficiency and Disease by Robert R. Barefoot --- 5th edition
Bibliography
Includes subjects:
1. Health and Ionized Calcium
2. Mineral Deficiency, Calcium Deficiency
3. Cancer and Calcium
4. Heart Disease and Calcium
5. Saliva pH and Calcium Body Fluid pH
6. Electromagnetism and Calcium
7. Digestion and Calcium
8. Calcium Chemistry
9. Calcium and Cancer
10. Allergy and Calcium
11. Medical Misinformation
12. Recipes for Good Health
13. Recommendations
14. Calcium and Allergy
Library of Congress Catalog Card Number, C.I.P.   92-90529
ISBN 0-9633703-2-4
Manufactured in Canada by Webcom Limited

Table Of Contents

Endorsements

"Mr. Barefoot is one of the Nation's top Nutritional Therapists, a chemist, scientist in the fields of biochemistry, hydrocarbon extraction and metal extraction from ores, inventor and holder of numerous patents, public speaker, writer, and outstanding business entrepreneur, a man of great integrity, enthusiasm, determination, loyalty, and tireless energy, coupled with a great personality. Mr. Barefoot has achieved wide acclaim in recent years for his biochemistry research into the inter-relationship between disease and malnutrition, espousing that degenerative diseases are caused by mineral and vitamin deficiencies," Howard W. Pollock, Congressman (Alaska) Retired, Past President Safari Club International, Ducks Unlimited, and The National Rifle Association.

"I have been a practicing physician for the past 25 years. I am a fellow of the American College of OB-GYN and a diplomat of the American Board of OB-GYN. Mr. Barefoot has helped me immensely to understand the complex chemistry of how calcium and other minerals contribute to overall health and preventive medicine. I personally know of many individuals who are much healthier today because of Mr. Barefoot's nutritional advice, including myself.," Wayne Weber M.D., Family Planning Associates Medical Group Inc., Los Angeles, California.

"I am a heart surgeon at Westchester Medical Center in Valhalla, New York, one of the largest open-heart surgery centers in the United States. I have had a special interest in nutrition over the past 30 years and have lectured on this subject throughout the United States, particularly its relationship to heart disease and other degenerative diseases. It is in this capacity that I have come to know and respect Robert Barefoot. He is an internationally known chemist with numerous international patents. His use of bio-chemistry in the field of hydrocarbon extraction and the field of metal extraction of ores led him to pursue a different line of

ix

research over the past two decades, elucidating the intimate relationship between nutrition and disease," Richard W. Pooley, Professor of Surgery, New York Medical College, New York.

"I am a physician, President and Executive Medical Director of Health Insight, S..B.S. and Health Advocate Inc., in the State of Michigan. I have extensive credentials and honors that reach the White House and Heads of States in other countries. Mr. Robert Barefoot is a remarkable gentleman and a scholar who works endlessly to complete his mission to cure America. He has worked over the past 20 years with many medical doctors and scientists across the United States and in other countries doing Ortho-molecular Research on various diseases. The information has been culminated in two books, 'The Calcium Factor' and 'Death by Diet' which have been used technically as Bibles of Nutrition. Many people I know have thanked Mr. Barefoot for both saving their lives and returning them to good health. Mr. Barefoot is an amazing and extraordinary man who is on a 'Great Mission' for all mankind. I thank God for Robert Barefoot ", Liska M. Cooper, M.D., Detroit, Michegan.

"I am a physician practicing at the Molecular/Biological level for over 25 years. I lecture extensively in the nutritional-medical field in Canada, the United states and Internationally. I have attended hundreds of lectures and seminars covering the aspects of medicine including a number of those given by Robert Barefoot whose discourses easily classify as absolutely excellent ! Personal conversations with this man, a highly moral and ethical person, have served to confirm his unusual knowledge in the field of biologically applied nutrition and immunity enhancement." C.T. Taylor, M.D., L.M.C.C., P. Eng., Stony Plain, Alberta.

"I have been an attorney involved in very complex litigation involving natural supplements and their ability to treat or cure various types of illnesses, including cancer. I am a well known in Maryland as a litigater, repeatedly being named as one of the outstanding trial attorneys, specializing in complex matters of all

natures and have written concerning trial techniques. Mr. Barefoot was engaged as an expert in the use of natural supplements, specifically minerals, and their effect on various forms of cancers. He is a renowned author in this field. There have been many occasions when I found him to be extraordinarily knowledgeable in this field of expertise. My professional opinion is that Mr. Barefoot's knowledge and experience with minerals and other natural substances and their application for the treatment of illnesses is unique. In fact, I am not aware of any other individual who possesses the knowledge and expertise in this very important and expanding field as Mr. Barefoot," David Freishtat, Attorney, Freishtat & Sandler, Baltimore, Maryland.

"Mr. Barefoot has been, and continues to be, an advocate for health and natural healing through nutrition and knowledge. He has championed the cause of well over 440,000 American women and children who have been exposed to the toxic effects of silicone implanted devices. Mr. Barefoot, one of the rare silica chemists in the world, has delivered a message of hope to these suffering individuals, who didn't have any hope before, but are now arming themselves with the books **The Calcium Factor** *and* **Death By Diet** *and are spreading the word. The name Barefoot has become a household word. In the past three years, he has traveled to count-less meetings and medical conferences throughout the country without charging for his services. Robert Barefoot is a humani-tarian and his efforts to educate through his books, informational tapes, lectures and vast media appearances has set a standard of excellence that is well above the norm. His work with hundreds of scientists and medical doctors, researching diet, has elevated him to one of the top speakers on nutrition in the nation,"* Jill M. Wood, President Idaho Breast Implant Information Group, Boise Idaho.

"I recently retired as President and CEO of Bioflora Inter-national Inc., a manufacturer of nutritional supplements, liquid mineral extracts, and liquid organic plant foods. I oversaw the formulation and production what is considered the world's best selling mineral supplement. I was originally introduced to and very

*impressed by the work of Robert Barefoot, specifically **The Calcium Factor** in 1996 but was not afforded the pleasure of a personal introduction until 1998. By that time he had developed a reputation and a title, "The King of Calcium,"* G. Scott Miller Past President & CEO, Bioflora Phoenix, Arizona

"I graduated from Harvard University in 1942 (BSc Chemistry) and worked as a Research Director and in corporate management, Franklin Electronics Inc., and have been awarded two patents. Mr. Barefoot has been highly influential in my survival of prostate cancer, with which I was diagnosed in the fall of 1991. Because of his detailed knowledge of biochemistry, he has much more penetrating knowledge of the relationship between disease and nutrition, a knowledge not available to many trained dieticians because of their lack of biochemical background. With his expertise, he has aided me in not only arresting the progression of my disease, cancer, through diet and nutrition, but also reversing it. Mr. Barefoot is, simply put, an extraordinary individual," Philip Sharples, President Sharples Industries Inc. Tubac, Arizona.

"I have known Bob Barefoot for three years during which time he has provided my spouse with critical information. As a result of this relationship, I was able to introduce dozens of people to Mr. Barefoot's idea relative to critical illness and nutrition. The results achieved have been remarkable. It is my personal opinion that Mr. Barefoot is the absolute top of his field, nutritional therapy," W. Grant Fairley, The Fairley Erker Group, Edmonton, Canada.

"I am a chemist and have been involved in product development, specifically nutritional supplements. I have written numerous articles and lectured throughout the United States on these products and the benefits of utilizing alternative medicine and alternative medical products within the U.S. healthcare regimen. Over the past three years I have traveled and lectured with Mr. Barefoot on numerous occasions all over the United States. He is recognized as a world class expert on calcium and its nutritional benefits for the human body. Mr. Barefoot blends his prestige and

uncanny ability to talk to the average person in a way that allows complicated scientific subjects to be completely understandable and accepted. I have seen Mr. Barefoot's information help a lot of people," Alex Nobles, Executive Vice President, Benchmark USA Inc., Salt Lake.

"I have been associated with Mr. Barefoot since 1993. His Nutrition therapy is the result of twenty years of research into non-invasive treatment of generic diseases. In Canada we now have six M.D.'s practicing his protocols. I understand that numerous Russian M.D.'s in Moscow are also practicing his protocols. This number will increase exponentially as the testimonial success of hundreds of afflicted people becomes known. Mr. Barefoot's biochemistry and science brings credence to his recommended dietary and lifestyle protocols. He must be considered at the top of his field," Peter Epp. P. Eng., President Albritco Development Corporation, Calgary, Canada.

"I am the General manager of an audio cassette tape manufacturer. Previously, I was the Vice President of an engineering consulting company specializing in nuclear technology analysis under contract to the U.S. government. With a BS degree in Electrical Engineering, graduate school work at UCLA and over 10 years of research at McDonnell Douglas, my technical and scientific tools are extensive. I currently specialize in the audio production of technical information specializing in nutrition and health. It is in this regard that I have come to know the reputation and work of Robert Barefoot. Our company actively seeks men and women with scientific and medical backgrounds in order to develop substantive resource material for our client base. Robert Barefoot's lectures, books and tapes support his position as a leading spokesperson for the benefits of nutrition for good health," Al Vendetti, General Manager, Exxel Audio Productions, Oceanside, California.

"I am the founder of a company that specializes in both mining and the export of health and nutritional products overseas. Mr. Barefoot has tremendous knowledge of biochemistry and his

expertise in the field of calcium research has earned him recognition worldwide for both his lecturing and his research. He has authored several books which my company exports overseas as nutritional standards for people involved in the nutrition industry. He has also researched and developed calcium supplements, which are being exported to several countries abroad. His research of the relationship between disease and nutrition is gaining recognition worldwide and if properly implemented, could substantially reduce the devastating effects of degenerative diseases caused by mineral and vitamin deficiency," Brett R. Davies, President, Davies International, Denver, Colorado.

"I am well known in the area of nutrition. I am certified by the National Association of Health Care Professionals as a Health Care Councilor and have lectured extensively in the United States, Canada, Russia and the Ukraine. Mr. Barefoot is considered one of the most knowledgeable people in the world, on effects of calcium on health", Robert G. Bremner, Mechanicsville, Virginia.

"Mr. Barefoot is a man in pursuit of" Excellence", in all his endeavors. He has received wide recognition for his research in the biochemistry field, dealing with malnutrition. I have the distinct privilege and pleasure of having known Mr. Barefoot for several years", Jerry R. Gallion, International Financier, Vaulx Milieu, France.

Foreword

The Calcium Factor was written to both inform and instruct the general public about one of the hottest topics of research in the scientific community: biological calcium. Each scientist specializes in his specific and complex arena of interest much like a musician specializes in his specific musical instrument. The purpose of this publication is to unlock the information hidden within scientific technical jargon contained within thousands of publications, and to demonstrate to the layman that all of the thousands of scientific arenas of research can easily be orchestrated using *"The Calcium Factor"* to produce an understanding of the symphony of life.

Calcium has also become a hot topic for nutritionists who are extolling its virtues in promoting good health. The general public is being told that "calcium is good for you" and food pro- ducers are responding by fortifying numerous products with cal- cium. Since promoting calcium is becoming old hat — just ask the dairy industry — then why another book on calcium? The answer is simple. **The Calcium Factor** explains with detailed technical mechanism just *how* calcium works, and also explains *why* calcium is superior to all other elements in performing the biological tasks that are required to prevent disease and maintain good health. Also, the critical link between calcium and vitamin-D will be discussed in detail, and daily consumption of these two critical nutrients will be recommended in amounts substantially higher than the Recommended Daily Allowance (RDA's). In doing so the book becomes controversial to orthodox medicine which, although it has an excellent track record in dealing with catastrophic illness, has a dismal record in both dealing with and accepting preventive medicine. **The Calcium Factor** was written to withstand scientific scrutiny and criticism. Criticism from those who benefit from the maintenance of disease only serves to endorse the importance of understanding calcium's role in nutrition, as historically, all great concepts that are currently accepted by those who criticize were initially vigorously opposed by their predecessors prior to their total acceptance by the world at large.

The historical resistance to change of the governing establishments in the scientific and medical communities, as well as the resulting negative effects on innovation and research, will be explained. Dr. Carl Reich will be shown to be one of these innovators who fell victim to the system. Quotes from world renowned scientists, including several Nobel Prize winners, will be given in support of the significance of the calcium factor to human health. A detailed explanation of the chemistry of calcium will be given to show how it has become the *king of the bioelements* or the common denominator of good health. All of the scientific and medical facts will be presented in an order that supports this *unified concept of disease*, with calcium being the *"silver bullet"* for many dreaded diseases such as heart disease and cancer. Using cell physiology and biochemistry, an explanation will be given to show that healthy body fluids are alkaline as is demonstrated by the bright alkaline blue saliva test for children and the healthiest athletes, and to show that the sick have body fluids that have become severely acidic, as is demonstrated by the bright acidic yellow saliva test for patients with terminal diseases, such as cancer which experts recognize *cannot survive in an alkaline medium.* Calcium deficiency will be shown to be directly correlatable to acidic saliva pH which is a reflection of the acidic state of the body's fluids. A scientific explanation will be given of how very moderate amounts of food supplements, in the form of vitamins and minerals, can regulate good health. Also, the influence of electrical and magnetic fields on regulating health will be explained in simple scientific terms.

Calcium makes up 1.6 percent of the human body weight, making it the most abundant metallic element. As such, it plays a myriad of crucial roles both structurally and biochemically. Only recently have scientists begun to unravel the intricacies that make calcium the *King of the bioelements.* They found that a drop in the level of calcium in the body is intricately involved in the process of aging as well as a host of degenerative diseases such as osteoporosis, allergy, gallstones, cancer, heart disease and many more.

The **Calcium Factor** explains *how* and *why* calcium plays such a pivotal role in human health while also explaining how the degree of acidity of body fluids, which can be simply measured by spitting on a penny's worth of pH paper, is directly related to the trigger of disease: *calcium deficiency.*

The **Calcium Factor** also explains how preventive medicine consisting of a change in life-style, accompanied by modest food supplements, can quickly overcome mineral deficiency, and in doing so can shoot down disease with the *the silver bullet, calcium.*

The most distressing aspect of medicine today is that the Recommended Daily Allowance (**RDA**) for minerals and vitamins, although ridiculously low and *disease-inducing* (the new **RDI's** will be set at half as much), is rigidly adhered to, even though our society is heading towards several medical disasters, as is witnessed by the staggering increase in AIDS and cancer. Although medicine is winning a few battles, it is definitely losing the wars. For example, in the 1950's cancer was striking one out of every four people; by the 1980's cancer was striking one out of every three people; by the year 2010 cancer will strike *one out of every two people*. AIDS is also skyrocketing with virtually no hope with the current medical approach of packaging a solution in a chemical drug. Since the AIDS victims do not die from the disease directly, but from other diseases that are able to attack their defence-weakened body, it makes sense that although a person may carry the virus, high pH body fluids may strengthen the body's health to the point where the disease is not allowed to flourish, as is the case with cancer.

Fortunately, the medical pendulum is beginning to swing in the opposite direction. There is a growing movement that wants to do more than just use chemicals and drugs to block the symptoms of disease. By researching biochemical processes, calcium deficiency has been shown to be the trigger for a whole host of diseases. The road to the prevention and the cure for these diseases can be found in the knowledge expounded in **The Calcium Factor.**

The scientifically defendable suggestion that diseases can be prevented and even cured nutritionally will most certainly be received by both skepticism and *medicine's traditional cry of "quackery"*. The authors hope that such is the case, as most major advances of medicine in the past have been greeted by the same chorus. For example, Dr. Ignas Semmelweis was run out of the medical profession for the "quackery" of advocating in 1847 that physicians wash their hands. More recently, the pioneers of electro-biochemistry who introduced the electro-encephalograph (EEG) to medicine, were called *"electronic quacks"* by the American Medical Association.

The examples given of the behavior of the medical and scientific communities are *historical facts*, and are not meant to demean either profession to which each author respectfully belongs. All criticisms are directed at the few in the upper echelon administrations of the governing bureaucratic establishments who rigidly regulate the innovation of doctors and scientists while vigorously protecting their own prestigious status quo empires. Unfortunately, criticism of these elite and most respected men is often met with the blind and defensive cry, *"blasphemy"*, thereby providing encouragement for the system to perpetuate its mistakes at the cost of human lives and suffering. Ironically, blasphemy is "the disrespect for persons or things regarded as sacred". This implies that such men are holy and therefore incapable of making mistakes. It is hoped that by our pointing out a few, the reader will be alerted to the fact that history may once again be repeating itself. More importantly, the implementation of the knowledge expounded in this publication, **The Calcium Factor**, could provide an innovative alternative for the frustrated physician and the disheartened patient.

Unfortunately, before the physician can practice preventive medicine, he must prove that nutritional therapy works to the satisfaction of the governing regulators who already have refused to examine the massive documentation available, most of which was provided by the world's best scientists, some of whom won Nobel Prizes for their efforts. In other words, the American Medical Association just refuses to listen to logic, preferring to tread the beaten path of escalating disease treated by unnatural and expensive man-made chemicals. The cost of this stance is massive human suffering, and the premature death of millions of Americans. The best remedy would be an *amendment to the American Constitution enshrining medical freedom*; thereby, allowing both doctors and patients the right to practice and to preach preventive medicine:

" Each and every American citizen has the right to choose and to practice the form of medicine that the citizen deems most beneficial to personal health, without economic, physical, political, or verbal interference or abuse, and any institution or governmental agency assigned to protect the state of the individual's health should be empowered only to make recommendations that do not infringe or prevent the individual's right to choose and to practice any form of medicine. "

However, amendments to the Constitution are very rare, and require years to succeed. The American public is desperate today, and cannot wait for this urgently needed change. Thus the best interim remedy would be for each state and the U.S. Congress to legislate an *Alternative Medicine Protection Act* to read as follows:

" A practitioner of traditional or alternative medicine, registered by an appropriate government authority, who engages in medical or nutritional therapy or in any relevant health procedure, including the recommendation or sale of health supplements, that departs from orthodox or conventional medical treatment, shall not be found to be unqualified, unprofessional, negligent nor guilty of assault upon a patient, nor be denied the right to pursue her or his professional practice or livelihood, solely on the basis that the therapy employed is an alternative remedy, or is non traditional or departs prevailing orthodox medical treatment, unless it can be conclusively demonstrated that the therapy has a safety risk for a particular patient unreasonably greater than the traditional or prevailing treatment usually employed for the patient's ailment. "

(Howard W. Pollock, Former Territorial Chairman of the Legislative Committee on Statehood for Alaska, and First Republican U.S. Congressman for Alaska.)

Preface

For over three decades, Dr. Carl Reich was known as a *medical maverick*, because of his choice to both practice and research preventive medicine. He contended that a nutritious diet that included dietary supplements, along with a healthy outdoor lifestyle could not only lead to a life basically free of disease, but could also provide an effective therapy and the means of preventing the occurrence of many of the so-called incurable diseases. Of course this would be almost impossible to prove, and therefore Dr. Reich was not considered to be a serious threat by the disease-dependent medical establishment, so he was left alone to do his task.

Almost immediately from the beginning of this practice in 1950, Dr. Reich recognized that most of the diseases his patients suffered from seemed to be directly correlated to what he suspected was calcium deficiency. He scoured the medical literature, not realizing at the time that most medical research trails behind scientific research by several decades. He was unaware of the importance that the scientific community was beginning to give to calcium in biochemistry, and therefore, for thirty years, had to fight the battle of ignorance alone and unaided. By changing the lifestyles of his patients and giving them mineral and vitamin supplements, he was able to turn their lives around. As word of his successes grew, his practice flourished. He tried to share the fruits of his research with his medical peers. However, they reacted by shunning him as if he had the plague. He continued to develop clinical procedures and to successfully treat thousands of grateful patients who had received no benefit from orthodox medicine, until finally, he had gone too far. While his patients all loved him, his medical peers began to complain, and so, after thirty-two years of successful practice, his license was suspended.

By 1964, Carl Reich had been practicing medicine for fourteen years, when an inquisitive young chemical student, Bob Barefoot, read an article that was to change his outlook on life. The article was about research of calcium depletion of the bones, and how this process paralleled aging. The article suggested that if the process could be slowed down, so too would the process of aging, thereby suggesting that the secrets of calcium could lead to the *"fountain of youth"*.

Mr. Barefoot became a chemist specializing in mineral digenesis, which is the process by which minerals are constantly changing from one form to another. Being an innovator, Mr. Barefoot researched and published scientific articles on the subject. He later began researching metal extraction in the mining industry, for which he attained international patents, and also researched enhanced hydro-carbon extraction in the petroleum industry. All the time he was doing this research he was also aggressively amassing technical publications that concerned biochemical calcium. Ironically, he found that, if he was to be successful in the mining and petroleum industries, an advanced understanding of the chemistry of calcium was necessary, as calcium is a major and active constituent in geology. Mr. Barefoot experimented with altering and creating calcium compounds and minerals, such as calcium phosphate (apatite), which is also the major constituent of bones. He found that to accomplish this within the hydrocarbon reservoir, chemically buffered solutions, much like the ones in the human body, had to be developed. Thus, over the years, Mr. Barefoot had amassed a great deal of advanced chemical knowledge and was up to date with the scientific community when he fortuitously, or by destiny, met the medically suspended Dr. Reich.

Mr. Barefoot had always had allergies, the most difficult being asthma. He had recognized as a young man that his asthma attacks were inversely proportional to his exposure to sun, or in other words, they did not occur often whenever he had a good tan. He later noted that the good health of his growing children seemed to directly coincide with their exposure to sunshine and nutritious foods. Thus, Dr. Reich's medical theories and observations, concerning vitamin-D and body calcium, paralleled many of his own scientific theories and observations. Mr. Barefoot quickly applied Dr. Reich's medical theories to note rapid and near complete relief of his own mild chronic sinusitis and his reoccurring asthmatic attacks. In turn Dr. Reich took support from Mr. Barefoot's scientific experiences. Both eagerly agreed to collaborate and share their theories and discoveries by writing a publication for the layman so that he and others could obtain relief from these and other allergic diseases and so that everyone could understand and share the joy of good health and longevity.

From the beginning Barefoot and Reich had a decided advantage over the scientific and medical communities, as they had proof that it was *the calcium factor* that was the key factor in preventing and curing disease. Thus, they simply had to examine the dietary habits of cultures that never got sick, and many of these cultures exist to this day. For example, it was well known, and documented, that the Eskimo culture never had degenerative diseases such as cancer and heart disease until the white man started feeding them. Also the Hopi Indians in Northern Arizona never got cancer, while cancer ravished all of the cultures surrounding them. However, it was decided that the scientific community would probably attribute the *gene factor* as the reason. Thus it was decided to look for larger and more distant cultures. An article in the January 1973 edition of **National Geographic** entitled *Search For The Oldest People* provided examples of many of these cultures including the Abkhasians from Georgia (high in the mountains), the Hunzas of Pakistan (high in the mountains), and the Vilcabambas of Ecuador (high in the mountains). This list was quickly expanded to include the Bamas in China (high in the mountains), the Azerbaijans (high in the mountains), the Armenians (high in the mountains), the Tibetans (high in the mountains), and the Titicacas of Peru (high in the mountains. To this list the Okinawans of Japan (sea level) were added.

With all of the above cultures, *disease does not exist:* no cancer, no heart disease, no diabetes, no Alzheimer's, no arthritis, etc. These cultures have no mental disorders and no doctors. They also live decades longer than we do in North America and their aging process is dramatically slower. The common denominator is that all of their water is loaded with mineral nutrients from melting glaciers high in the mountains, and from the disintegrating coral reefs in Okanawa. One quart of Hunza water contains 17,000 milligrams of calcium (17 times the RDA at the time), and they drink several quarts each day. In general, the over-riding factor in their disease-free longevity is the fact that these cultures consume almost *"one hundred times the RDA"* of everything. Also, they eat large amounts of everything we are told is not good for you such as butter, salt, eggs, milk and animal fat. Another major factor is that these cancer-free people are in the sun, which we are told causes cancer, most of the day. **The Calcium Factor** details the scientific explanations for their remarkable health and youth.

Acknowledgement

The authors are grateful and wish to acknowledge their appreciation for the dedication, contributions and efforts of Joyce Tiffin, Don McCormick, Philip H. Sharples, Marvin Livingston and Bruce and Carole Downey, and most of all, Karen Barefoot, in assisting the completion, critical review and editing of this publication.

Notation

Although this publication is intended to direct the attention of both the physician and the patient to the torrent of scientific research being carried out on the significance of biological calcium, it is not the intention of the authors to provide an alternative to the orthodox physician-patient relationship. Rather, it is the objective of the authors to expand the dimensions of orthodox medicine itself, and help speed it towards medical practices of the twenty-first century where diet and lifestyle will play a predominant role in preventive medicine.

"If the doctors of today do not become the dieticians of tomorrow, the dieticians of today will become the doctors of tomorrow." (Rockefeller Institute of Medical Research).

CHAPTER ONE

SCIENTIFIC AND MEDICAL TRENDS IN HISTORY

It is said that one of the most important reasons for learning history is because it repeats itself, and therefore to know history is to know the future. The reason for this phenomenon is that man is both a creature of habit and predictable emotions that preside over logic. Thus, we find that the trends in medical history both follow and parallel the trends in scientific history where many a genius has been destroyed by people of lesser talent defending the status quo. Therefore, before judging the medical innovator, it is necessary to put him in historical perspective so that our views are not clouded by the biased authoritarian establishment, whose track record, as you shall see, leaves a lot to be desired.

"Innovation is a twofold threat to the scientific hierarchy. First, it threatens their oracle authority. Secondly, it evokes the deeper fear that their whole laboriously constructed authoritarian edifice may collapse" (Arthur Koestler, **The Age of Velikovsky**).

1

In 1808, Dalton, the father of modern chemistry, proposed the "*Atomic Theory*", that atoms were the basic components of all substances. The scientific establishment of the day threw scorn on his theory. More than sixty years later, in 1869, Professor Williamson, President of the Chemical Society, "humored" those who accepted the theory stating that "*for lack of any better theory, it would have to do for now*". Even after one hundred years had elapsed, prominent scientists of the day, such as the renowned Professor Ostwald, were publicly administering scathing condemnations for Dalton's theories, while attempting to show that the theory of chemistry was independent of the theory of atoms. For other lesser known scientists of the day, such as Albert Einstein and Max Planck, the atomic theory was as correct and as natural as sunshine. In contrast, almost two hundred years later, almost every educated man in the world believes in Dalton's Atomic Theory.

Albert Einstein, who was unquestionably the most famous scientist of the twentieth century, had to withstand more efforts by the establishment attempting to disprove his theory of relativity than has ever been made to disprove any other theory in the history of science. This was demonstrably shown by one of his opponent's publications entitled *One Hundred Against Einstein*, to which he remarked that "*if they were right, one would be enough*".

Max Planck, a father of modern physics and Nobel Prize winner in 1903, stated that "*An important scientific innovation rarely makes its way by gradually winning over and converting its opponents; it rarely happens that Saul becomes Paul. What does happen is that its opponents gradually die out and that the growing generation is familiarized with the idea from the beginning.*"

And so, despite the uphill battle, road blocks, and mine fields maintained by the scientific hierarchy of the day in an attempt to defend their prestigious status quo, science managed to progress to the point where, by the 1950's, the scientific establishment arrogantly announced to the world that "*in this atomic age, all there is to know has already been learned and all future advancements would be simply rearrangements of current knowledge*". The old adage, "*The more we know, the less we know*" was certainly not believed by this incredibly arrogant group of scientists.

While all these impediments were being placed on progress in basic science, medical science was also experiencing similar resistance to progress. For example, in 1841 Ignas Semmelweis, a Hungarian physician who was horrified by the high death rate of women giving birth in hospitals, became obsessed with finding the cause of the disease. At that time mothers who had given birth at home or in carriages on their way to hospital had a far greater chance of surviving their childbirth than if they had been delivered in a hospital. Moreover, in that period it was common practice for doctors to go directly from the morgue, where they conducted post mortem examinations and anatomy classes using the bodies of deceased patients, into the maternity ward and attend maternity patients dressed in usual garb, without washing their hands. For these and other reasons, Dr. Semmelweis suspected that the doctors were carrying an agent on their hands that was causing the fatal disease. In 1847, Semmelweis instituted a procedure of scrubbing and dipping the hands in a chlorine solution before every procedure, the death rate fell from *thirty percent to practically zero*. The protective medical establishment of the day reacted by blocking Dr. Semmelweis's application for research funds and proceeded to vilify, ostracize, and finally have him discharged from his prestigious positions in maternity hospitals. Haunted by the fact that hundreds of thousands of women continued to die, Dr. Semmelweis eventually died of insanity in 1865. By the 1880's, the advent of the microscope made the invisible microbe visible, and doctors began to universally adopt Semmelweis's procedures. Despite the

3

eventual acceptance of the hand scrubbing technique in maternity wards, both Louis Pasteur and Joseph Lister encountered great difficulty in having the *germ theory of disease and antiseptic surgery* accepted because the leading physicians of the day adamantly refused to accept the theory.

A few years later, Theodore Boverie, the true father of genetic science, discovered almost every detail of cell division including chromosomes which, he concluded, transmit heredity. This idea was strenuously opposed by the protective establishment, led by Thomas Morgan. Years later, Morgan found that his own experiments agreed with Boverie's. Quietly disregarding his previous criticism of Boverie, Morgan went on to describe the chromosome structure in more detail adding specific positions called "*genes*", for which he received the Nobel Prize in 1937.

While all this research was going on, a few brave scientists were attempting to correlate the existence of bioelectrical systems with biological functions. Traditional biologists were horrified, and were, for the most part, successful in removing the funding for such experimentation. The medical establishment was likewise so miffed by these proposals that it was determined to block the propagation of such nonsense. Even under this severe duress, electro-biochemistry was further researched and when the pioneers of "electro-encephalography", the recording of electrical brain impulses referred to as an *EEG*, employed the new procedure, they were called "*electronic quacks*" by the American Medical Association.

More recently, electro-physiologists such as Dr. Robert Becker, a research orthopedic surgeon, found, as others had before him, that he had to wage a constant battle against the "*frozen thinking of the establishment*", who to this day continue to block the results and advancements in this field. One such example is the natural ability of children under puberty to regenerate chopped off fingers and toes when the skin is not sutured over the stump but is only dressed to allow the exposed tissue to remain electrically negative, a practice carried out in many hospitals outside North America. In fact most Western doctors refuse both to believe these results. Likewise, acupuncture, a safe and natural procedure for pain suppression, is supposedly accepted by the medical profession, but practiced only in limited fashion. Instead, doctors continue to kill over 50,000 Americans each year with anesthetics. By ignoring the fact that most biological functions are electrically controlled, the medical profession remains ignorant to the fact that the low frequency electromagnetic fields, generated by most of the electronic or electrical gadgetry of our day, will superimpose over these natural bioelectric fields, thereby altering their functions. The result is a host of potential medical problems. This type of *"electropollution"* will become common knowledge to every child in the twenty-first century. However, back in the twentieth century, the doctors did not understand how a pulsed magnetic field from an electric appliance could possibly affect the health of his patients. Also, although it is difficult for a Western physician to understand how a needle inserted in the head can cure a pain in the stomach, as is done by the Eastern physician, he readily accepts that a pill in the stomach can cure a pain in the head. True logic will only prevail once the best of both worlds is permitted by the always intransigent medical cartels.

How does the intelligent, highly educated well-trained physician of today find himself in the same head-in-the-sand ostrich position that was adopted by his medical regulators? The answer is simple. His profession, like that of the scientist, is one of the most extremely regulated professions in the world. In addition, his time is largely consumed in attending to his patients and, as he is sensitive to the opinions of his peers, he succumbs to total control by his regulators, on whom he has become basically dependent for survival in this calling. There can be no doubt that each practitioner is quite eager to apply any new technology that is

5

endorsed by his medical superiors in teaching and research institutions. There can also be little doubt these elite few have a vested interest in maintaining the status quo of ignorance. Their actions moreover are whole heartedly endorsed by the powerful drug, military, and electrical utility establishments, all of whom have a vested interest in maintaining economic control. Thus, just as scientific advancement is suppressed by the scientific hierarchy of the day, so too, the advancement of medical science is suppressed by the medical hierarchy. History teaches us that this system has been in effect for hundreds of years, with the individual scientist or doctor participating as an innocent and ignorant victim of the system.

Unfortunately, the general public of the day has also been purposely kept uninformed, and thinks of the medical profession in *"God-like"* terms. After all, each generation is impressed by the spectacular advances in medicine that are applied to challenging very limited selected areas of medicine, while the majority of the public remain silent victims of the untreatable diseases that affect the masses. A well planned public relations program results in a favorable public reaction to *"the great scientific advances of modern medicine."* However, to put these advances in perspective, one must imagine taking a *time trip* back in time to visit the busy doctor of one hundred years ago. To your horror, a scruffy doctor would begin to treat you with dirty, unwashed hands, probably just after he had finished an autopsy. Anesthesia had been recently discovered and surgery was becoming popular; for an abdominal complaint, after a little blood letting, the physician would recommend a *"go in blind and find"* solution to your problem. Then, if you bled too much during the surgery, a lethal transfusion of un-typed blood would probably be administered. If you managed to survive, you, a time-travelling member of an advanced generation, would probably scream at the doctor to *"change his archaic procedures"*. This would result in the medical authorities of the day having you incarcerated, but only after you had first been humiliated and vilified.

Another enlightening time-travel trip would be for someone from a future generation, say one hundred years from now, to return to Earth to visit one of our current busy doctors conducting his practice today. The time-traveler would be astounded by the *"factory medicine assembly-line"* approach that was devoid of the *"preventive medicine"* approach with which he was so familiar. In surgical practice, particularly in the treatment of cancer, he would be mortified by the *"cut it and cure it"* approach that was supplemented by *"burning it out"* with radiation. He would be equally disturbed by the use of noxious and harmful chemicals for the pain induced by these barbaric procedures. He would be astounded by the laboratory testing that most always resulted in the recommendation of synthetic drugs. Moreover, he would be distressed that, despite advanced research that was being done at the time, the physician almost never recommended that the ill or seriously diseased patients change their lifestyle, including diet, and take dietary supplements. In frustration, the time-traveler would scream at the doctor to both change his archaic procedures and begin to apply the knowledge of nutrition that prevailed and to use the painless and non-destructive electro-physiological techniques that were being pioneered at the time, to thereby begin investigating all the possible means of treating and preventing the occurrence of disease.

Thus, the trends of history are the same as human nature, never changing. *"Great spirits have always encountered violent opposition from mediocre minds"* (Albert Einstein), and *"Resistance to innovation is clearly demonstrated, not by the ignorant masses, but by professionals with a vested interest in tradition and the monopoly of learning"* (Arthur Koestler, **The Age of Velikovsky**). The frustrated innovators, working not in establishment orientated institutions, but at the grass roots of science and medicine which is the logical source of practical innovation, unfortunately, must all follow the same path. And so it was for Dr. Carl Reich, who, after a lifetime of discovery, innovation, and medical practice during which he satisfied thousands of grateful patients, found himself suspended by the medical authorities. His "*crime*", after thirty-four years of practice without one patient complaint, was the pursuit of the practice of **Preventive Medicine**, which included revolutionary, therapeutic advances employing *"The Calcium Factor"*. Dr. Reich was also chastised by the medical authorities for his claim that *"calcium can cure cancer"*, as well as several other degenerative disease. A claim which they believed was to simplistic to have any medical credibility, and a claim which two decades later would be triumphantly published and endorsed in medical establishment's own journals (See Chapter Sixteen)

CHAPTER TWO

HEALTH AND
IONIZED CALCIUM

Over one hundred years ago, the calcium ion in blood serum was discovered to be a significant factor in maintaining the contractility of the heart. This accidental finding was the important base from which much of the focus on biological calcium originated. When Dr. Reich began his medical practice in 1950, there were about *50 publications* per year by the scientific community on biological calcium. By 1990 the number had exponentially swollen to over *7000 publications* per year, with medical researchers joining the biochemical researchers. From the very beginning of his practice, Dr. Reich had recognized the significance of biological calcium, and had instituted a clinical research program in which he developed procedures and tests that allowed him to gain both clinical and statistical proof of the key role that the calcium ion played in human health.

The human body is made up of all the most common elements in the world (see Table 1, page 35) with the exceptionof silicon and aluminum. Although all these elements are required to sustain life as we know it, in the final analysis, the presence

9

of no one element can be said to be more important than any other element. However, what can be said is that some elements are more abundantly intertwined in the vast array of bodily functions than are others. Therefore the abundance of these elements is crucial to the maintenance of good health and to life itself. Through its natural evolution over many millennia the body developed a survival defense mechanism which compensates for any changes in the concentrations of these elements. Excess elements are readily expelled from the body. Deficiencies, on the other hand can only be partially overcome by the induction of biochemical reactions through the adaptive functions of organs in an attempt to best balance this loss. The result is *a physically weakened body that is prone to disease of these adapting organs*.

One of the most important of these integral elements is the element *calcium*. It can be found molecularly bound in the bones in abundance, and in almost all human cells. When freed from its molecular bonding by ionization, it can then readily combine with proteins. The inclusion of such calcium bound protein in the ion channel on every cell wall constitutes biological valving that regulates both cell nutrition and the important bioelectrical cellular discharging processes involved in all bodily functions. Vitamin-D, produced in the skin by a chemical reaction induced by the ultraviolet radiation of sunlight (photosynthesis), has as its main function, the ionization of ingested calcium by the small intestine. Although the inside walls of the small intestines are very negatively charged, the positively charged ionic minerals have a hard time being absorbed *"through"* the intestine walls. Fortunately the walls of the small intestine contain vitamin-D receptors or VDR's, which allow the long chain vitamin-D to *penetrate deeply* into the intestine wall and leave its negatively charged oxygen end exposed at the surface. This allows the positively charged calcium ion, and other positively charged ions, to latch on to the negatively charged oxygen on the end of the vitamin-D and be drawn into and through the intestine wall. It is estimated that filling the VDR receptors with vitamin-D allows the body to absorb up to 20 times more calcium. Thus *photosynthetically produced vitamin-D* (lots of sunshine) and/or vitamin-D supplements are crucial to the absorption of nutrients. At the same time, photosynthesis also results in the production of *inositol triphosphate, INSP-3*, which serves to regulate the extraction of calcium stored in the cells. This process is triggered to supply the cell with calcium when insufficient calcium is ingested and ionized by the Vitamin-D process. If there is insufficient calcium stored within the cells, then the parathyroid hormone, stimulated by the deficiency of Vitamin-D, induces the *extraction of calcium from the bones*. Finally, with bones severely weakened by this calcium depletion, the body beings to extract its ionic calcium from the proteins that are regulating cell functions. The resulting cell dysfunction's manifest themselves with a whole host of symptoms and diseases identified correctly by Dr. Reich as the "*ionic calcium deficiency syndrome and diseases*", but most doctors know them only as chronic disease of unknown or obscure origin.

Sufficient ingested and ionized calcium can therefore not only prevent many diseases, but due to its involvement in cell nutrition, it can also maintain vigorous good health. Calcium's involvement in cell nutrition is three-fold. First, as mentioned, calcium bound proteins regulate both the size and the opening and closing of the ion channels of every cell wall. Secondly, the calcium ion, substantially more than any other ion, has the capability of attaching itself to a large number of nutrient radicals, which are molecularly stacked on the outer surface of the cell membrane. When these "*stacks*" become electrically detached (detailed discussion of this process will be given in chapter five) the calcium ion is capable of transporting them through the cell ion channel thereby delivering the most amount of nutrients for the healthy function of the cell. Thirdly, calcium combines with the phosphates in the extracellular and intracellular fluids to create a slightly alkaline, buffered and oxygen rich medium necessary to sustain life. *Only the element calcium* is capable of creating and maintaining these critical conditions.

With such a vital role to play in human health and with all the currently massive amount of research being carried out by the scientific community one would think that the medical profession would eagerly grasp the importance of "the calcium factor". However, as history has taught us, the medical profession has not been quick to respond to simple concepts, such as washing their hands, so the concept of the true importance of milk and sunshine supplements to good health should be equally as difficult for them to accept. In addition, history has also shown us that it takes the medical profession several decades to accept new and proven scientific advances.

In 1950, there was only a minor amount of interest by the scientific community in the mechanisms involving calcium in the human body. In contrast, almost immediately after beginning his practice and clinical research, Dr. Reich recognized that a whole host of symptoms such as indigestion, headaches, and muscle pains, and of diseases such as chronic arthritis, ileitis, colitis and asthma, were caused by an overall *calcium deficiency* in the body. He also reasoned that vitamin-D was *crucial* to the absorption and utilization of calcium, and that, since man's mode of living had evolved from a loin cloth to a tuxedo, the amount of vitamin-D produced from exposure to sunshine had diminished dramatically. He also recognized that, nutritionally, man's consumption of calcium and other critical elements was deficient and had to be increased. He therefore recommended changes in diet and life-style to his patients, and prescribed supplementary calcium and vitamin-D. The results in improving the health of his patients were both quick and dramatic. Eager to share these exciting results, he approached his medical peers, only to find that, as other innovative doctors before him had found, he was to be *shunned for his unorthodox practices*.

12

For decades, Dr. Reich continued to assess and to treat the ionic calcium state of his patients. He did this by studying their lifestyle, diet, physical complaints, and their *inter-relationships to various diseases*. He treated thousands of grateful patients who were either dissatisfied with, or had not received benefits from orthodox medicine. All the while he amassed a large amount of data in his clinical studies, and became more and more convinced that caring about the health of his patients was far more important than caring about criticism from the medical elite, or pursuing scientific *"double blind"* studies that they demanded. Their demands were also accompanied by income restrictions, hospital access denial, and refusal of research grants.

It was not until the early 1970's that Dr. Reich further discovered that *the acidic state of saliva was an outstanding manifestation of calcium ion deficiency*. This was extremely important as it meant that by simply measuring the pH of the saliva with inexpensive litmus paper, a three second test, the basic state of health of the patient, in reference to calcium ion deficiency, could be determined. He found that when a patient was non deficient in calcium and healthy, the pH of the saliva was slightly alkaline at 7.5 to the neutral pH 7.0, and the body excretions tended to be acidic. But, when the patient was ionic calcium deficient, the salivary pH was acidic, from 6.4 to 4.6, and the body excretions tended to be alkaline. In addition, he found that patients who were developing physical ailments tended to be in the 6.5 to 6.0 pH range, with those who already were showing serious ionic calcium deficiency disease most frequently showed a pH below 6. After only a few weeks to months of dietary changes along with vitamin and mineral supplements, he noted that the saliva pH would slowly rise up to 7.0, and the physical impairments would dramatically improve or be eliminated.

Unfortunately, because of the weakness in human nature that resists innovation and because of the simplicity of his medical approach, in 1984 the medical authorities rewarded his efforts by examining his fitness to practice and by the cancellation of his *license to practice medicine.* During this thirty seven years of practice, not one complaint had been received from any one of the thousands of patients he had treated. On the contrary, his patients were extolling the virtues of this new approach to medicine. Also during this period, the scientific research publications on *the calcium factor* in the human body had increased from a trickle to a torrent. Although interest by the scientific community in calcium has been dramatically raised, interest by the medical community remains at nothing more than idle curiosity. Thus, remembering that medicine takes decades to adopt scientific discovery, and that *Medical Freedom* does not exist in America, history had once again repeated itself.

Today, mankind is in dire need for the medical profession to study and apply the knowledge contained in the horde of readily available scientific publications so that they will be better able to understand the effects of the calcium factor on human health, and to begin participating in this advancement in medical science. By using the simple clinical tools developed by Dr. Reich, they could begin the time-journey from the twentieth century's mode of treating disease with drugs to the twenty-first century's mode of *preventing disease nutritionally.*

CHAPTER THREE

QUOTABLE QUOTES

When statements are made that are obviously very controversial, some means of measurement must be found in order to gauge the merits of the arguments. Since the importance of calcium as the "*king of the bioelements*" is a scientific argument, then statements by respected men of science, by their sheer numbers and emphatic conclusions, should convince any unbiased third party. Unfortunately, those involved in judging the argument are prejudiced by a vested interest in maintaining the status quo, and that is why the famous Max Planck said that the next generation will be allowed to accept the new concepts as soon as the older establishment *"gradually die out."*

In the previous two chapters, a number of statements were made that the medical hierarchy may consider false and without foundation. The references to history refer to facts that *can be confirmed* in any public library. References to statements on the *calcium factor* are supported in both scientific research publications and books. The following constitutes several of many quotations made by renown researchers:

"The Prime Cause and Prevention of Cancer", Otto Warburg, Lecture at the meeting of Nobel Laureates, June 30, **1966** Director, Max Planck Institute for Cell Physiology, Berlin.

"There is no disease whose prime cause is better known, so that today ignorance is no longer an excuse that one cannot do more about prevention of cancer. But how long prevention will be avoided depends on how long the prophets of agnosticism will succeed in inhibiting the application of scientific knowledge in the field of cancer. In the meantime millions of men and women must die of cancer unnecessarily." (Note: in 1966 cancer struck 23% of Americans, whereas today it strikes 39% of Americans).

"Breathing Easy", by Lendon Smith, M.D., in the book **Feed Your Kids Right**, Dell Pub. Co. Inc., **1979**.

"Calcium is required all our lives for bones, teeth, muscle, nerve function, and for blood clotting. Muscle pains, cramps, twitches and even convulsions may suggest calcium deficiency."

"For asthma, 1000 milligrams of calcium should be given daily along with 1000 units of vitamin-D for intestinal absorption. Calcium can relax the muscles surrounding the bronchial tubes while altering the permeability of the cell walls, allowing the nutrients to get in."

"How a Mineral Can Vitalize Your Health", by Dr. James K. Van Fleet, in the book **Magic of Catalytic Health Vitalizers, 1980,** Parker Publishing.

"According to nutritional authorities, the American diet is more lacking in calcium than in any other essential food. Dr. Henry C. Sherman, the noted biochemist, has stated in effect that **the prime period of human life could be extended by a moderate increase in calcium** *in the diet. It would also be wise to get at least 400 units of vitamin-D daily to insure proper absorption of the calcium from the tract into the body where it can be utilized."*

"When the body does not get enough calcium, it will withdraw what little calcium it has from the bones to make sure there is enough in the bloodstream, then the body does its best to bolster the sagging architecture by building bony deposits and spurs to reduce movement and limit activity."

"Calcium in Synaptic Transmission", by Rodolfo R., **Scientific American**, October **1982**.

"The connection between the electrical activity of the cell and the release of the neurotransmitter is not direct; an essential intermediary is the calcium ion."

"The Role of Calcium in Biological Systems", Volume I, **1985**, CRC Press Inc.

As a prelude to the quotations in this book, the following comments, contained in the brackets, are made to help the reader better understand the quotations: (**The Role of Calcium Biological Systems** is a compilation of dozens of scientific publications by academically recognized scientists. This book deserves particular note because world class scientists are *concluding* that there is a link between calcium deficiency and cancer. Also, the hundreds of scientific references contained in this book, as well as the other books quoted, could lead the reader to thousands of scientific publications on the importance of biochemical calcium. Although the first quote is self-explanatory, the second quote may be difficult for the reader to understand. Basically, it says that calcium deficiency in the body fluids outside and inside of the cell *stimulates the proliferation* of both virus and cell mutation (**cancer**) by regulating DNA synthesis. Furthermore it concludes that calcium deficiency is the universal property of *all* cancer cells, the knowledge of which may be *the key to understanding cancer*.

The biochemical mechanisms that trigger and stimulate cancer will be explained in detail in Chapter Eight, *Calcium and Cancer*).

"Calcium must certainly be the major bioelement of the times. Only a generation ago the calcium ion was known to physiologists and biochemists as a component of bone mineral and as a blood plasma constituent required in heart function and blood coagulation, but little more. But, in the 1970's a crescendo of calcium ion research developed. Today we know dozens if not hundreds of different cellular and extracellular processes that are regulated by the changes in cytosolic or extracellular calcium ions. Indeed, the calcium ion is emerging as a most important and ubiquitous intracellular messenger" (Forward, Albert Lehniger, Professor of Medical Science, John Hopkins University).

"As we have seen, calcium is central to the ordered progression of replicating cells through their growth- division cycle. Neoplastic epithelia and mesenchymally derived cells can initiate DNA syntheses and proliferate normally in a low calcium medium, which does not support the proliferation of their normal counterparts. Besides needing calcium ions, normal cells must adequately spread out on a solid substrate before they are able to initiate DNA syntheses Calcium is specifically required for spreading. Lowering the extracellular calcium and preventing spreading both block the initiation of DNA synthesis, without stopping on-going DNA synthesis. The elimination of extra- cellular calcium requirement for proliferation of viruses can be mimicked by exposing proliferatively inactive calcium-deprived normal cells to calcium-independent-nucleotide protein kinases located in the plasma membrane. Thus, addition of such subunits to the medium of normal cells cause them to behave like neoplastic cells by initiating DNA syntheses in calcium deficient medium. It is clear that the proliferative calcium independence in vitro is a universal property of neoplastic cells, the understanding of which may be the key to understanding cancer." (page 158, Volume #1)

"Calcium Homeostasis: Hypercalcemia and Hypocalcemia", **1986**, Gregory R. Mundy, Professor and Head, Division of Endocrinology and Metabolism, University of Texas.

*"A number of **important metabolic processes** are influenced by small changes in extracellular ionized calcium concentration. These include; (a) the excitability of nerve function and neural transmission; (b) the secretion by cells of proteins and hormones, and other mediators such as neurotransmitters; (c) the coupling of cell excitation with cell response (for example, contraction in the case of muscle cells and secretion in the case of secretory cells); (d) cell proliferation; (e) blood coagulation, by acting as a cofactor for the essential enzymes involved in the clotting cascade; (f) maintenance of the stability and permeability of cell members; (g) modulation of activity, in particular those enzymes involved in glycogenolysis, gluconeogenesis, and protein kinases which are calcium dependent; and (h) the mineralization of newly formed bone."*

"Calcium in the Action of Growth Factors", by W.H. Moolenaar, L.K. Defize, and S.W. Delaat, **1986 Calcium and the Cell**, 1986, Wiley.

*"Proliferation of cells in vivo is regulated by polypeptide growth factors. Binding of growth factors to their specific cell-surface receptors initiates a cascade of biochemical events in the cell which ultimately leads to **deoxyribonucleic acid (DNA) synthesis and cell division**. The immediate consequence of receptor activation include a sustained increase in cytoplasmic pH and a transient rise in cytoplasmic free calcium ions. The platelet derived growth factor induced calcium ion signal is due to calcium ion release from intracellular stores, whereas the epidermal growth factor seems to activate a voltage independent calcium*

19

*channel in the plasma membrane. These results suggest that the rise in calcium ions is **indispensable for cell proliferation**."*

"Calcium and Cell Function", Volume VII, Wai Yui Cheung, **1987** Academic Press Inc.

*"The regulation of mitosis and cell division is one of the fundamental questions of cell biology. Calcium has been **implicated as a regulatory factor in both**."*

*"**History of Calcium-Binding Proteins**"*, in the book **Calcium Binding Proteins**, by Marvin P. Thompson, CRC Press **1988**.

*"Calcium has been recognized as a **major regulatory ion in all living organisms**."*

*"Considering the wide variety of calcium binding proteins in the cell, **the potential targets of calcium-related disorders are enormous**."*

*"General interest in calcium binding proteins is still in the **logarithmic phase** with daily discoveries of these proteins.*

"Intracellular Calcium Regulation", Felix Bronner, **1990**, Wiley.

*"One of the astonishing developments in biological research is **the recent widespread interest** in the role played by calcium in cellular metabolism."*
"Intracellular calcium regulation will be of interest to researchers and graduate students in the areas of biochemistry, biophysics, cell rheology and nutrition."

"The Green Leaves of Barley", Dr. Mary Ruth Swope, **1987**, Swope Enterprises Inc., P.O. Box 62104, Phoenix, AZ 85082-2104. 1 (800) 447-9772

"There are many research studies which allude to the fact that high phosphorus and/or phosphoric acid (found in meat and soft drinks) pulls calcium out of the bony structures (bones, teeth and nails) in the process of digestion and assimilation. This has a **disastrous effect on bone density,** *leaving them porous and spongy. When calcium is pulled from the bones, it is released through the kidneys, resulting in* **stone formation** *(kidney stones) before it is excreted."*

"The Calcium Signal", **Scientific American**, November **1987**, by Ernesto Carafoli and John T. Penniston:

"A **common trigger precipitates biological events** *as diverse as the contraction of a muscle and the secretion of a hormone. The trigger is a* **minute flux of calcium ions.**"

"To control cellular process effectively, calcium itself must be regulated. Knowledge of these intricacies (elaborate system of proteins that interact with the calcium ion regulating intracellular messages) may lead to greater clinical control over intracellular calcium, a possibility that has **broad implications for the treatment of disease.**"

"The Calcium Connection", Dr. Cedric Garland and Dr. Frank Garland, **1989**, Foreside, Simon and Shuster Inc.

"Low cancer areas were far more frequent in the sun belt. (This statement is contrary to the incorrect popular belief that sunshine causes cancer). *What was the significance of sunlight with regard to cancer rates? Sunlight reacts with cholesterol*

inside and on the surface of the skin to create vitamin-D. Vitamin-D helps the body absorb calcium and plays a major role in the body's ability to use the calcium that is available."

"Treatment of Vertebral Osteoporosis", by Dr. Meunier in the book **Molecular and Cellular Regulation of Calcium and Phosphate Metabolism, 1990** Alan R. Liss Inc.

*"When calcium and vitamin-D is given in daily doses along with moderate amounts of sodium fluoride to patients with osteoporosis, there is a substantial increase in bone mass and a **significant reduction** in the incidence of further vertebral fractures."*

"Calcium Takes Its Place As a Superstar of Nutrients" Jane Brody, October 13, **1998**, New York Times.

*"Calcium is fast emerging as the nutrient of the decade, a substance with such diverse roles in the body that virtually no major organ system escapes its influence. A research team at the University of Southern California in Los Angeles reported in The American Journal of Clinical Nutrition that adding calcium to the diet lowered blood pressure. Dr, Susan Thy-Jacobs, a gynecologist at St. Lukes Roosevelt Hospital Center in New York believes that "a chronic deficiency or imbalance of calcium is largely responsible for the disruptive symptoms of PMS suffered by women". Dr. Martin Lipkin of the Strang Cancer Research Laboratory at Rockefeller University in New York said that "Animal research indicated that increasing calcium levels to protect epithelial cells from cancer might also help **prevent cancer** in such organs as the breast, prostrate and pancreas".*

"Calcium's Powerful, Mysterious Ways", Jennifer Couzin, May 3, **1999**, U.S. News & World Report.

*"Researchers are increasingly finding that the humble mineral, calcium, plays a **major role** in warding off major illnesses from high blood pressure to colon cancer. You name the disease and it's beginning to have a placed there,"* says David McCarron, a nephrologist at the University of Oregon Health Sciences University in Portland. *"In the past year, calcium has also been reported **to reduce premenstrual symptoms, and it may protect against heart disease.**"*

Since there are thousands of scientific publications on biological calcium, thousands of more quotes could be given supporting the crucial role of calcium in human health. However, in just the few that were given, statements by the most prestigious scientists in America have explained *how calcium is **responsible for cell division and cell growth**, and how calcium deficiency is **the key to cancer** and other degenerative diseases.*

In all of these statements made by these scientific and medical researchers, there is one common denominator, that is that they are all ***adamantly convinced*** about the importance of cellular calcium or the ***Calcium Factor*** in the state of human health. While thousands of scientific publications have been written in support of their convictions, thousands more are being prepared for the press. The research has gone from its first historic stage where the initial theorists were both inhibited and scorned by the scientific hierarchy, to the second stage where it now is not only academically acceptable to pursue this work, but a few others in the medical profession are beginning to experiment. The third state or research will occur when the medical hierarchy begins to enthusiastically support this research, and finally the fourth state will begin when the medical profession at large enthusiastically begin to apply the ***Calcium Factor*** in their daily treatment of the these theories beyond doubt, is that mankind has to suffer the painful and needless wait. As two time Nobel Prize in Medicine winner, Otto Warburg stated, "As long as the agnostics succeed in inhibiting the application of scientific knowledge in the field of cancer, millions of men and women must die of cancer unnecessarily" (1966). While the orthodox doctor both cures and kills with the painful procedures of the twentieth century, Dr. Reich and others like him have cured with the painless procedures of the twenty-first century, as *no patient was ever killed by implementing a healthy change in lifestyle,* including diet supported by moderate dietary supplements and vitamins.

Hippocrates who lived from 460 to 377 BC, was known as the *"father of medicine"*. Orthodox doctors who take the *Hippocratic Oath* and who depend on man-made, and therefore unnatural, chemical medicines should note that Hippocrates believed that "the body has a tendency to *naturally heal itself* and that *"food is the best medicine and the best foods are the best medicines"*.

Note:

1.   DNA or deoxyribonucleic acid, referred to in many of the quotes, is the double-strand helix structure discovered by James D. Watson and Francis H. Crick in 1953, that carries the information that cells need to build and organize proteins for healthy cell growth. Dr. Reich was well into his medical practice prior to the discovery of DNA.
2.   For the purpose of emphasis, the author has italicized key phases in some of the quotations.

CHAPTER FOUR

SUMMARY OF SCIENTIFIC RESEARCH

Throughout the time when Dr. Reich was conducting clinical research on the calcium factor, he was thoroughly up to date with the few medical publications in his area of research. However, he was *unaware* of both the growing importance that the scientific community was placing on the same subject, and the advances in scientific knowledge that were lending support to his hypotheses. Thus, a summary of this work is in order.

Although the quotes from some of the research being done on the calcium factor can provide some insight into these scientific advancements, they provide little or no information as to how these advances apply to your personal health. The information is *locked within the technical jargon* in the masses of available literature. However, there would be no doubt in your mind, once you began to review the massive amount of research being done, about the significance that so many prominent scientists place on the importance of calcium in the human body. What is required before this technically garbled information can be put to use is for someone to present a total overview of the research in layman's terms. This would require a summary of the research by the scientific community that is followed up by integration with medical observations, and then, finally, recommendations to employ this knowledge about *the calcium factor* to maintain good health. In this chapter, a summary of some of the pertinent scientific research shall be dealt with.

At the beginning of this century calcium was known by biologists and physiologists to be a component of bone material, and little else. Then it was discovered as a necessary constituent of blood plasma required in blood coagulation and heart function. Only a few, such as Baird Hastings, Walter Heibrunn and Carl Reich, saw more clearly into the future of the calcium ion as a total body health factor, a future that would be a long time coming.

From the beginning of Dr. Carl Reich's medical practice, he began by immediately recognizing that many of the medical ailments of which his patients were complaining, were accompanied by what he suspected was *a deficiency in ionized calcium*. Dr. Reich had long since recognized that the increased frequency of such ailments seemed to parallel the basic change in lifestyles brought on by the comforts and diet of the time. The most notable change was *the exposure to sunshine*, or rather the lack of it, by the modern urban dweller. He noted that *patients who did have significant exposure to sunshine, usually did not demonstrate the same severity of these ailments* included the dietary considerations in his analysis, with special consideration to the consumption of foods rich in the alkaline minerals, mainly calcium, *almost all of his patients fell into three classes;* 1) those with both significant exposure to sunshine and dietary consumption of large amounts of calcium and vitamin-D rich food (ie: fish) who did not exhibit the chronic diseases of the time, 2) those who were exposed to lesser amounts of these commodities who exhibited various symptoms, and 3) those who were more severely deficient and who experienced one or more of a variety of these diseases and their symptoms.

Dr. Reich reasoned that *the common denominator of these symptoms and diseases was a deficiency of dietary calcium, dietary vitamin-D, and of sun-on-the-skin production of vitamin-D* which is *an absolute requirement* for the intestinal absorption of digested calcium. Without the effect of adequate vitamin-D from one or both of these sources, he reasoned that most of the consumed calcium would simply pass through the body. The logical recommendations to his sick patients, *a change in their lifestyle with dietary supplements of vitamin-D and calcium*, made Dr. Reich a maverick amongst his peers, and a hero to his cured patients.

To his utter astonishment, this simple and successful approach was not only rejected by his peers, but was also frowned upon by the medical authorities. They would not support these dietary supplements claiming that *there may be harmful side effect*s, this despite the fact that, while people were dying with these ailments, *no one ever died from the vitamins and supplements* taken in the moderate dosages that Dr. Reich was recommending. These were about the amounts that a person would ingest and produce in their skin when eating an optimal diet and being outside in the sunshine daily. Despite these successes, his arguments fell on deaf ears. This was the "*super scientific*" nuclear age; how something so simple could have any merit, was the question that doctors asked as they methodically scrubbed their hands before operating on their next patient, a patient who was probably suffering from calcium deficiency. Needless to say, the matter was further complicated by both the way Dr. Reich's practice flourished, thereby undoubtedly introducing the further problem of professional jealousy, and by the resistance that Dr. Reich made to the restrictions that were arbitrarily placed on his practice by medical committees, boards and councils.

Before describing Dr. Reich's studies and clinical research in detail, it is important to overview the parallel scientific research on the importance of biological calcium that was being carried out by many who have been *recognized as world renowned scientists*.

The first significant work was done in the late 1950's and early 1960's by A.L. Hodgkin and A.F. Huxley, for which they won a *Nobel Prize in 1963*. They researched and measured the means by which the nerve cell membrane is electrically charged and discharged. Although the calcium ion was not integrated as part of their research, it was later shown by other researchers to play an integral role in these processes. Hodgkin and Huxley showed that the electrical excitability of the nerve membrane depends on its possession of a voltage sensitive ionic permeability system. This enables it to utilize energy stored in the ionic concentration gradients set up by an energy-dependent ion pump.

In order to understand this system, it is first necessary to understand that the interior nerve cell and its axon, or nerve fiber, as well as most other types of living cells, is rich in potassium, while the body fluids outside are rich in sodium. In the resting state, the exterior membrane is much more permeable to potassium than to sodium, (an energy dependent ion pump driven by the hydrolysis of ATP, *adenosine- triphosphate*, selectively pumps more potassium than sodium into the cell) resulting in the retention of much more potassium within the cell and much more sodium outside the cell. This causes an electrical potential difference with the inside of the cell to be in the 70 millivolt-range between the two surfaces.

Hodgkin and Huxley postulated the existence of parallel sets of ion channels that were selective for sodium or potassium, and were controlled by the electric field across the membrane. The event that triggers the electrical activity of the nerve is a *depolarization of the membrane*, that is, a reduction of the potential difference or voltage across it. This depolarization opens channels or pores in the membrane, with a mechanism that was not understood at the time, allowing sodium to flow into the cell. The wave of depolarization shoots down the nerve fiber triggering either muscle reaction or some other important biological function such as stimulation of the secretory cells.

Hodgkin and Huxley theorized that it was the size of the opening of the ion channel that selectively allowed the ions to migrate through, potassium being much larger than sodium. It was only much later that the actual mechanisms of both the triggering mechanism and the ion channel valving mechanism was much more thoroughly understood. In both cases, calcium ions played the pivotal role. Therefore, *a deficiency in calcium ions would have serious consequences to the transmission of nerve stimulus, muscle movement, hormone secretion, and other important biological functions*.

In the 1970's the scientific world witnessed *a crescendo of biological calcium research*. Hundreds of different cellular and extracellular processes, that were regulated by the changes in the level of extracellular calcium were researched. At least three different membrane systems of the cell take part. Remarkably, it was discovered that extracellular calcium levels can regulate several different cellular activities simultaneously, raising fundamental concerns about the regulations of cellular fluid calcium ion concentrations, especially when the body is overall calcium deficient. Researchers also found it remarkable that both calcium and phosphate occur in the extracellular fluid and urine in supersaturating concentrations, but *do not precipitate into stone*. They reasoned that some biochemical mechanism prevented this from occurring.

In 1982, Rodolfo R. Linas, while researching calcium in synaptic transmission (synapses are the junction sites at the tips of the fibers that sprout from each neuron or brain cell) was able to explain how a current of calcium ions *triggers the passage of signals from one nerve cell to another*, the process of electrical nerve stimuli. He found that a neuron at rest has a potential difference of 70 millivolts between the inside of the cell and the outside. The depolarization which is caused by the energy of physical stimulus, is not sufficient in itself to cause the release of a transmitter. Depolarization is the means by which an inward current of calcium ions is induced to flow through the membranes to the synaptic terminal, which is similar to a secretory process.

In addition, Linas found that *a supply of calcium ions must be present in the extracellular environment for depolarization to occur*. Linas found that in every secretory process, the secretion is triggered by an increase in the concetration of calcium inside the secretory cell. The calcium could only come from the external environment or from internal cell stores. Therefore, just as a deficiency of calcium in the system would affect the production of secretion, the release of neurotransmitters would also be affected.

Linas assumed that the potential difference or voltage between the inside and the outside of the synaptic terminal was created by the difference in the concentration of calcium ions across each cell membrane. Each cell membrane contained calcium pores or channels through which *"a rosette shaped"* set of five proteins extended. Each rosette was created by a large *calcium binding* protein molecule. Increasing the voltage between the outside and the inside of the membrane resulted in a stretching, or an uncoiling, of the rosette or valve, thereby allowing more calcium ions to enter the cell. Thus, this calcium binding of proteins produced a system to regulate the influx of ions through channels into the cell. The "*unknown mechanism*" of Hodgkin and Huxley was therefore finally explained.

By 1985, Carafoli and Penniston had further studied the importance of the calcium ion in controlling biochemical processes. They found that a "*common trigger*" precipitates biological events as diverse as the contraction of a muscle and the secretion of a hormone; the trigger is *a minute flux of calcium.*" They described the array of proteins that are specialized to bind calcium creating the molecules that serve to regulate the concentration of calcium ions within the cell as well as mediating its effects. They also found that these calcium bound proteins were essential to the role of ionic calcium as an intracellular messenger. Some of the calcium bound proteins control calcium concentration in the cell, thereby producing electrical signals, while others serve to receive the signals.

By 1986, Moolenaar, Defize and Delaat had found that a sustained increase in cytoplasmic pH and a transient rise in the free calcium ions in the cytoplasmic cellular fluid was a necessary function of DNA synthesis and cell division, stating that "*the rise in calcium ions is indispensable for cell proliferation.*"

By 1988, Marvin P. Thompson, in summarizing the work done to that date stated that "*calcium is a major regulatory ion in all living organisms, interest in calcium is in the logarithmic phase, and calcium related disorders are enormous.*"

By 1990, although thousands of publications and books had been written extolling the importance of *the calcium factor* in the human body, few dared to recommend the practice of clinically employing the knowledge gained, as Dr. Reich has done. Although the importance of cellular pH and calcium deficiency has been scientifically proven, medically, the jury is out! The jury is composed of the *old guard who, as history teaches us, have a vested interest in protecting the status quo, no matter the cost in human lives*. Unfortunately, just as Dr. Semmelweis had to do, Dr. Reich is also being forced to stand idly by and watch as thousands of patients die painfully and needlessly. Both men used *logic too simple for their peers to believe*; both men were ostracized by their superiors; both men were before their time.

(Note: In the October 1996 issue of **City Scope**, a well read magazine in Calgary Canada, a feature article *Ahead of His Time* was published in which Dr. Carl Reich was referred to as *The Father of Preventive Medicine* in tribute to his pioneering efforts).

CHAPTER FIVE

THE CHEMISTRY OF CALCIUM

One of the most important questions to be answered is why Calcium out of all of the elements on Earth, became the most important biological element of our times ? The answer can be found in the understanding of the basic chemistry of both calcium and deoxyribonucleic acid, DNA For those who are not amateur chemistry buffs, skip to the last paragraph in this chapter for the layman's summary.

Calcium is a metallic element with a density of 1.55 a valence of 2, an atomic weight of 40, and an atomic number of 20. Although lime was prepared by the Romans in the first century under the name *"calx"* the metal was not discovered until 1808, the year Dalton proposed the *Atomic Theory*. After learning that Berzelius and Pontin had prepared a calcium amalgam compound, Davy was able to isolate the metal for the first time. Calcium forms more than three per cent of the earth's crust, the fifth most abundant. It is never found in nature uncombined and occurs abundantly in the carbonate form as limestone, in the sulfate form as gypsum, and in the phosphate form as apatite. Chemically, calcium is one of the alkaline earth elements as its oxides react with water to form stable hydroxides which are basic: pH greater than 7. It has a low attraction for electrons and is a good reducing agent, that is, it gives up its electrons readily, especially to oxygen. The oxides and hydroxides are polar, that is, electrically charged oppositely at each end of the molecule. Calcium has 20 electrons with 2 in its outer fourth orbital. Its ion is the same size as sodium, bigger than magnesium, but smaller than potassium, all of which are very common.

What does all this mean? Let us simplify the basic physical characteristics that would be required by the bioelement with the job of participating in almost all biochemical functions, as well as providing basic structural building material that can readily be removed and replaced.

To begin with, it would have to be abundant; the most common elements in the earth's crust are oxygen at 49%, silicon at 26%, aluminum at 7.5%, iron at 4.7%, calcium at 3.4%, magnesium at 1.9%, hydrogen at 0.88%, titanium at 0.55%, phosphorous at 0.12%, carbon at 0.09%, manganese at 0.08%, sulfur at 0.03%, and all others at less than these elements (see Table#1). Although the elements of lower concentration than those listed cannot be ruled out, the chemically active element required would be more appropriately found with a higher range of concentration.

Table #1:   Elemental Composition of the Earth's Crust Versus the Human Body

Element	% Earth's Crust	% Human Body
Oxygen	49.00	65.00
Silicon	26.00	trace
Aluminum	7.50	trace
Iron	4.70	1.00
Calcium	**3.40**	**1.60**
Sodium	2.60	0.30
Potassium	2.40	0.40
Magnesium	1.90	0.05
Hydrogen	0.88	10.00
Titanium	0.55	trace
Chlorine	0.19	0.30
Phosphorus	0.12	0.90
Carbon	0.09	18.00
Manganese	0.08	0.00
Sulfur	0.03	0.25
TOTAL	**99.46**	**100.00**

Note: All other non-man-made elements (77 elements) make up 0.54 % of the earths crust.

It should be noted that all of these elements can be found in the human body, and the one that is lowest in concentration in the earth's crust, carbon, is the basic building block element of life as we know it. However, it is basically only a *"structural"* component, and must be chemically compounded with the element hydrogen in molecular form to be an active "functional" ingredient in the body. This compounding renders carbon less reactive, as it must always be attached to one or more hydrogen atoms, than the simple element that would be required for diverse biochemical activity.

The most abundant element, oxygen, is also never found unattached in its elemental form. It has six electrons in its outer second orbital, and is very aggressive in trying to fill up this orbital with two more electrons. This trait is known as *electronegativity*, and oxygen is number one in aggressiveness. The giving up or sharing of electrons resulting in elemental bonding, by definition, represents a chemical reaction. As a rule, elements with outer orbitals that are less than half full tend to give up these electrons, and elements with outer electron orbitals more than half full tend to acquire electrons to fill this orbital. Thus, oxygen preferentially binds itself to elements with outer orbitals not only less than half full, but also with the most available electrons. The list of most abundant elements with less than half full but that have the most electrons in their outer orbital for oxygen to "*grab*" are as follows: sulfur with six electrons, phosphorous with five electrons, silicon and carbon with four electrons, aluminum with three electrons, iron with three or two electrons, magnesium and calcium with two electrons, and sodium and potassium with one electron. Since the stability of the molecules formed depends on the number of electrons shared, and since oxygen is an integral part of life as we know it, we must remove the elements to which oxygen will most readily attach. Thus sulfur, phosphorous, silicon, carbon, and aluminum must be removed from the list of elements which were contenders for the most active biochemical element.

This leaves sodium, potassium, magnesium, and calcium as the most logical contenders. It should be noted that sodium and potassium are alkali metals, and magnesium and calcium are alkaline earth metals, or in other words, these elements all exhibit the physical property of producing alkaline solutions, pH greater than 7, when exposed to water. Thus it would be logical that most of the body fluids, in which the biochemical activity occurs with one or more of these elements, should have a pH greater than 7. However, the higher the pH of the fluids rise above 7, the more corrosive they become, and although certain restricted parts of the body, such as the stomach, can contain corrosive acidic fluids, every cell throughout the body definitely cannot. Both sodium and potassium produce very caustic and corrosive solutions and must be balanced with anions, such as chlorides, to bring their pH down to approximate neutrality at pH 7. On the contrary, both calcium and magnesium produce mildly alkaline solutions with a variety of anions, and thus require less dependence on the presence of other specific ions. Although all of these last four elements will be found to be important for body functions, *calcium and magnesium appear to be emerging as the most flexible*.

Another trait that would be desired would be *biological efficiency*, or in other words the ability of an ion to attach to a larger number of nutrient polar radicals or proteins. There are a large number of polar molecules, the most common being water (see diagram #1), and glucose. When under the influence of a strong electrical field, such as the negative cell surface mostly made up of phospholipids (see diagram #2), the polar compounds tend to stack themselves by having their oppositely charged ends face each other, creating the stack (see diagram #3). Since the outer end of this aligned stack is negative, the negative cell surface has thereby propagated its electrical field out to the end of the stack, where, at this point it can attach itself to a cation (positive ion). Both calcium and magnesium ions have two electrons missing from their outer orbitals which allows them to attract more of the polar stack extending out from the cell surface, thus emerging once again over sodium and potassium ions which have only just one electron missing from their outer orbitals.

Diagram #1: Polar Water Molecule with its Electrical Field

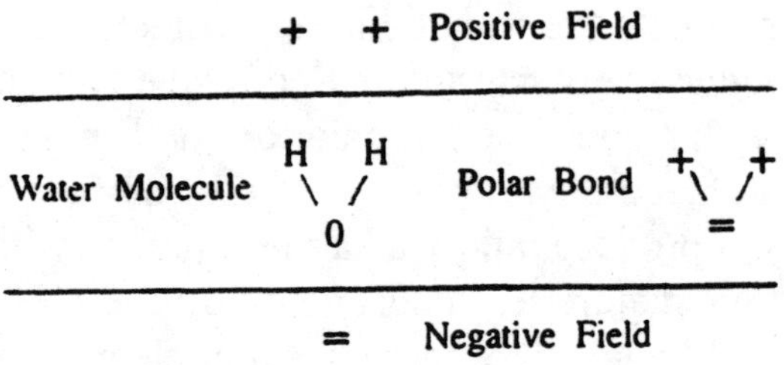

```
                    +    +    Positive Field
_____
                       H   H                        +    +
Water Molecule          \ /        Polar Bond        \ /
                         0                             =
_____
                    =    Negative Field
```

Diagram # 2: Phospolipds on Cell Surface With Its Negative Electrical Field

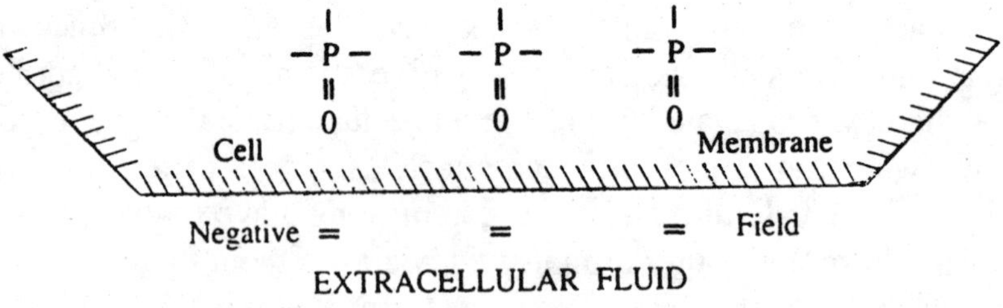

```
          |          |          |
         - P -      - P -      - P -
          ||         ||         ||
          0          0          0
     Cell                        Membrane

    Negative =         =         =    Field
            EXTRACELLULAR FLUID
```

Diagram #3: Negative Field Propagated Out from the Cell Membrane by Stacking Polar Compounds

$$-P- \quad -P- \quad -P- \quad -P- \quad -P-$$
$$O \quad\quad O \quad\quad O \quad\quad O \quad\quad\quad O$$

Cell | Membrane

Negative ... Field

Extracellular ... Fluid

POLAR ... STACK

Negative Propagated ... Field

Positive ... Cations

Ca   K   Na

$$\overset{=}{O} \quad \overset{=}{O} \quad \overset{=}{O}$$
$$\overset{\|}{-P-} \quad \overset{\|}{-P-} \quad \overset{\|}{-P-}$$

Ortho ... Phosphates

This process of electric field propagation is very common in nature and can be better understood by providing a simple illustration: dry sand readily pours out of a bucket when turned upside down; however, when a bucket of wet sand is turned upside down, the sand comes out in one whole piece, retaining its shape. This occurs because a particle of sand, like the phospholipid cell surface, is made up with oxygen on its surfaces. When wet, the polar water stacks up from all of the surfaces, thus propagating the negative fields outwardly until they meet and try to repel each other from all sides, resulting in each sand grain remaining suspended with enough force to defy gravity. This is similar to the two like-poles of magnetic levitation repelling each other to defy gravity thereby allowing a train to remain suspended in mid air. With the water-suspended sand, the crystals on the edge are prevented from being pushed off the stack by the force of the water surface tension. Similarly, this electric field propagated out from the cell is a strong force in organizing the positively charged cation *biochemical workhorses, such as calcium*. The most common polar compounds in the extracellular cell fluid are water and glucose. Sodium, potassium, calcium and magnesium cations are all frequently affected by this electrical field propagation, with other cations less frequently affected; however; once the stack breaks from the membrane, one element, *calcium*, is vastly superior in assisting nutrients into the cell .

Another ability that the master biochemical element must have is *the ability to readily release the stacked polar nutrients* once they have entered the cell. Magnesium has two electrons in its outer third orbital, while calcium has two electrons in its outer fourth orbital, and also has eight electrons with ten vacancies in its inner third orbital. Thus, because of its larger size and electron vacancies, calcium's electrons are much more loosely bound than are magnesium's, thereby allowing calcium to more readily give up its electrons to proteins and to polar nutrients. For example, calcium has a greater ability than magnesium to cross link with other molecules. *Calcium can bind to seven oxygen locations on a protein while still holding onto a water molecule*, while magnesium can only bind to three oxygen locations on a protein while holding on to two water molecules. The water molecules exchange at a rate five thousand times greater, and therefore much more easily, for calcium than for magnesium. Calcium is a larger ion than magnesium, therefore it *moves faster*. Calcium binds to the central atom of biologically important coordination compounds, ligands, both *ten thousand times as fast and ten thousand times as strong* as does magnesium. Since all of these abilities give calcium *the most chemical flexibility* to carry out the myriad of biological duties required to sustain life, *"calcium"* can rightfully claim the title of *"King of the Bioelements "*.

Of course there are many other reasons why calcium predominates so readily over the other elements in biological importance. It has been known since the time of the Romans as a strong building material, with much of the calcium in the cement *being both removable and replaceable without the structure collapsing*. This is also one of the most important properties in the human body, and as we shall see discussed in later chapters, while calcium is considered to be the biological glue that keeps all of the cells in the body from coming apart, much of it can be removed or replaced without breakup of the structure. Another important property, that has been discussed in the research literature, is calcium's ability to *behave like an octopus and bind to several different elements at once*, enabling it to bind and bunch up long proteins, an ability necessary to regulate entry of ions into the cell. Since ionization is required to produce a voltage that will regulate entrance through the cell membrane, calcium comes out the winner as, to produce a specific voltage, it requires the least of ionization. For example, 70 millivolts of potential difference between the outer and inner layer of cell membrane can be produced by the ionization of only 507 parts per million of calcium, while 933 parts per million of potassium would be required to produce the same voltage.

And last but not least, calcium also has the unique ability to form a soluble (mono) orthophosphate, which, in combination with calcium bicarbonate, acts as a *crucial component of a pH buffer system* that holds the extracellular fluid in the 7.4 pH range. Also, as calcium bonds to the phosphates, it liberates sodium and potassium, allowing them to form alkaline salts (which is discussed in Chapter 7 in more detail), as well as combining with bicarbonates to produce mild chemical buffers such as sodium bicarbonate in the pH 7.7 range. This alkaline pH buffering mechanism is crucial in allowing glucose to break down into the four nucleotides — *adenine, guanine, cytosine and thiamin* — that are the basic building blocks of DNA. When the pH drops below 6.5, becoming acidic, the glucose breaks down into lactic acid, thus creating even more acidity and starving the cell of the basic building materials it requires for DNA replication.

In summary, calcium is one of the most abundant elements on Earth. It is small enough to have the mobility to enable it to pass through small openings, yet it is large enough to have enough electrons in enough orbitals to influence a variety of bonding with other nutrient compounds. However, it has significantly less electrons in its outer orbital than most of the other common elements, thereby minimizing its entrapment with the most common element, oxygen. Calcium is the basic ingredient responsible for producing strong cellular building materials while retaining the ability to be removed and replaced without causing the collapse of the structure. Very little calcium ionization is required to produce necessary biochemical voltages. Calcium is the only element that can produce the crucial buffered pH of 7.4 required to DNA synthesis. Calcium is clearly the *King of the Bioelements.*

CHAPTER SIX

CALCIUM AND DIGESTION

Ironically, for a nutrient that is so necessary for the biochemistry of the body, calcium is one of the more difficult elements for the body to digest and absorb. Other compounds in most foods, such as phosphates in red meat, tend to keep it from being chemically broken down and dissolving. Moreover, once some calcium has dissolved, its absorption into the body is totally dependent on the presence of vitamin-D in the intestine. Unfortunately, vitamin-D is rare in most foods. Its intestinal concentration depends on being fortified by the action of the ultra violet band of sunlight on a fatty substance in the skin to synthesize vitamin-D. Insufficient intestinal vitamin-D results in *preventing sufficient calcium absorption into the body* in the ionized state that is crucial to so many biological functions. These factors make the digestion and absorption of calcium one of the most difficult tasks in nature.

According to the dictionary definition, "*digestion*" is the preparation of food for assimilation, or absorption into the system, in the stomach and bowels. In more technical terms that means the ionization of animal and plant nutrients, into their basic anion and cation components, so that these ions can be absorbed by the body.

The process of ionizing plant, animal, or mineral nutrients begins with pulverizing them through chewing and the action of the stomach to expose as much of the surface as possible to water. For some nutrients, such as the salt sodium chloride, the exposure to water is all that is required to initiate immediate ionization. Most nutrients, however, require the addition of acid to the pulverized nutrient and water mixture, to effect any significant amount of ionization. In order to understand this process more thoroughly, it is first necessary to understand just what an acid really is.

The dictionary defines an acid as one of a group of substances that neutralize or are neutralized by alkalies. This definition may help to class a group of substances, as either acids or alkalies, but for the average person, it does not explain what either substance truly is. The chemical dictionary defines acid as one of a large class of chemicals that has the property of ionizing or splitting of the water molecule, H-O-H, to produce positive hydronium ions, more commonly referred to as hydrogen ions, (H)+. In contrast, an alkali is a chemical that splits water producing the negative hydroxyl ion, (OH)-. Thus, acids are substances that ionize to give a solvent an excess of the positive hydrogen ion, and alkalies are substances that ionize to give a solvent the negative hydroxyl ion. The concentration of these ions, acidity and alkalinity, are described as numbers, pH values, that are logarithmic (to the base ten) reflections. When the number of alkaline (OH)- ions present in a fluid equals that of the acidic (H)+ ions, the fluid is in the neutral state and its pH is 7.0. Increases in acidic (H)+ ions produce changes from 7 to 0, while increases in alkaline (OH)- ions produce changes from 7 to 14. It is important to remember that the intervals on the pH scale are exponential. Therefore the pH scale represents vastly wider differences in concentration than the figures themselves seem to indicate. A pH change of one unit reflects a ten-fold change in the hydrogen ion or the hydroxyl ion concentration. This is evident from Table 2.

Table 2: pH

(H)+ Description	pH Value	Ratio of Concentration
	0	10,000,000
	1	1,000,000
Acid Side	2	100,000
Excess of (OH)+ Ions	3	10,000
	4	1,000
	5	100
	6	10
----------> Neutrality ---- --------->	7	----------------> 1
	8	10
	9	100
	10	1,000
Alkali Side	11	10,000
Excess of (OH)- Ions	12	100,000
	13	1,000,000
	14	10,000,000
		Ratio of (OH)- Concentration

It is therefore apparent that ionization occurs in both acidic and alkaline solutions, and although digestion in animals occurs in the acidic range, it is possible to have digestion occur in the caustic range, such as the digestion of feces in lime water. However, all human digestion is acidic. Fortunately, or by design, the digestive system is made more efficient by the fact that most foods are acidic, thereby generating their own acids and thus requiring less acid from the body for total digestion. Some examples are given in the Table #3.

Table 3: Food and pH

Food	pH
Lemons	2.1
Vinegar	2.7
Apples	3.1
Grapefruit	3.1
Rhubarb	3.1
Strawberries	3.2
Raspberries	3.4
Tomatoes	4.2
Bananas	4.6
Carrots	5.1
Beans	5.5
Bread	5.5
Asparagus	5.6
Potatoes	5.8
Butter	6.3
Corn	6.3
Shrimp	6.9
Water	7.0
Egg Whites	7.8

During digestion, hydrochloric acid is produced in the stomach and the gastric contents range from pH 1 to pH 3. Since almost all chlorides are soluble, that is, they remain ionized, the hydrochloric acid is a most effective way of ionizing the food. However, food usually contains products that produce ions other than chlorides, such as the phosphates from meat and soft drinks, the citrates from fruits, and the lactates from milk, to name but a few. When some of these anions are present in large numbers they present a problem, as they can bond together with other ions to create insoluble precipitates, which therefore are not ionizable at the strength of the acid that is in the stomach. An example of this is the precipitation of calcium phosphate, a mineral called "apatite", when the negative phosphate ion comes in contact with the positive calcium ion, with the resulting apatite being excreted from the body. If however, other anions, such as lactates from milk or malates from apples, are present in sufficient quantities, the calcium would form significant amounts of calcium lactate and calcium malate, which are both extremely soluble, and thereby remain ionized. This does not mean, however, that *just because the food is ionized that it will be absorbed by the intestines*. For example, as previously stated, vitamin-D is an absolute requirement for *the absorption of ionic calcium by the body*. Thus, without vitamin-D, most of the ionized calcium would pass through the body.

It is therefore apparent that eating the food which contains a nutrient that the body craves is not enough to maintain good health. Unfortunately, other pertinent parameters exist that will create an unhealthy state of the body even though apparently nutritious foods are consumed. An example of this is eating fruits and vegetables to get the trace metals that the body craves, only to remain deficient because the particular soil, that was chosen to grow these seemingly nutritious foods, was *barren in these required trace metals*. And finally, when the body consumes, digests and absorbs almost all of the nutrients it requires, (see Tables #4 & #5) but is deficient in only calcium, the body remains in an unhealthy state because the body's cells will not be able to fully utilize these nutrients. These mechanisms will be discussed in the next chapter. Thus, the consumption, digestion and absorption of foods rich in calcium and the provision of vitamin-D in the diet by the exposure to daylight and sunshine are necessary to maintain good health. (See Chapter 14: Recipes for Good Health)

Table 4: Original Major Nutrients in the Body

Nutrient	Weight %
* Water	39.10
Oxygen	20.30
* Glucose	19.10
* Methane	13.80
* Ammonia	2.90
Calcium	1.60
Iron	1.00
Phosphorous	0.90
Potassium	0.40
Sodium	0.30
Chlorine	0.30
Sulfur	0.25
Magnesium	0.05

Total	100.00

* Made up of the following elements

Oxygen	65.0 %
Carbon	18.0 %
Hydrogen	10.0 %
Nitrogen	2.4 %
Note:	95.4%

The chemical breakdown of glucose and the chemical combination of oxygen with methane results in the production of **34.6 %** more water, making a total of **73.7% water in the human body**

Table 5: Major Nutrients in the Blood (pH 7.3 - 7.5)

Component	Milligrams per 1000cc (ppm)*
Sodium	1400 --- 1430
Chloride	1000 --- 1040
Triglyceride Fat	950 --- 1050
Iron	950 --- 1000
Glucose	850 --- 1000
LDL Cholesterol	600 --- 1300
HDL Cholesterol	450 --- 850
Calcium	97 --- 106
Total Protein	72 --- 75
Potassium	40 --- 43
Phosphorus	31 --- 35

* ppm stands for parts of nutrients in the blood per million parts of blood.

CHAPTER SEVEN

THE CALCIUM CYCLE

Once the food has been digested and absorbed into the body fluids, the question arises as to how the nutrients get from these fluids outside the cells (extracellular fluid) into the fluids inside the cell (intracellular fluid) where they can be used for cell growth ? How is this flow regulated ? How are the nutrients con- verted to life sustaining electrical energy ? How does calcium play a role as the key ingredient to the answers to all of these questions ?

First, a brief description of a cell. It is the structural unit of which body tissue is made. Although it varies greatly in size, most are too small to be seen by the naked eye.

The cell is composed of an outer membrane (4 millionths of an inch thick) which encloses water-based fluids which contain billions of molecules that make up the biological components, such as enzymes, nutrients and DNA just to name a few. The interior of the cell provides a liquid medium for the breakdown of the nutrients providing both the energy and the biological building blocks necessary for growth. The nutrients and ions enter the cell through microscopic channels or pores and then the ions leave the cell through even smaller pores to continue the cycle. The cell surface membrane is capable of wrapping itself around and swallowing large components that it requires, a process known as endocytosis. The same process is reversed to expel large components it no longer needs and is called exocytosis.

As mentioned in Chapter 5, one of the key ingredients of the extracellular fluid is *calcium (mono)orthophosphate* which is extremely soluble in water, and helps buffer the pH at 7.4. A buffer is a solution to which moderate amounts of either strong acids or bases may be added without causing any large change in the pH value of the solution. As was also explained in **Chapter 5**, the surface of the cell is made up of phospholipids giving it a negative charge to which all of the polar nutrients, the main one being glucose, may be electrically stacked with their positive pole attracted to the negative phospholipid cell surface. This leaves the negative pole propagated out and away from the cell surface. The positive cations, such as calcium and sodium, attach themselves to the top of the stack where the negative charge from the polar stacking has been propagated. The positively charged cations do not totally eliminate the propagated negative charge as phosphates, rich in oxygen, also remain attached to the cations, leaving a net negative charge at the upper ends of these polar stacked nutrients. As was discussed in **Chapter 6**, a solution with a pH of less than 7 is positive and a solution with a pH greater than 7 is negative. Thus, the *extracellular fluids, with a pH of 7.4, are negative*.

Hundreds of scientific publications have been written describing the cell membrane ion channels or pores that allow entry of nutrients into the cell. Because of size, each channel is restrictive to specific ions. For example, a channel just big enough for sodium to enter would readily allow the smaller magnesium ion to pass, but would not allow entry to the larger calcium ion and the much larger potassium ion. These selective ion channels can be used to allow ions within the cell to exit, as the ions entering the cell are usually attached to large numbers of nutrient radicals and therefore require much larger channels. These large nutrient channels contain a *rosette of five proteins* each of which are bound in seven oxygen locations by the king of the bioelements, *calcium*. This causes the protein to bunch up, creating a plug that will shut off entry through the channel. As the nutrients within the cell undergo chemical reactions liberating their radical components that are to be used for cell growth and DNA synthesis, the attached calcium and other cations are also liberated. This production of cations inside of the cell drops the pH from 7.4 to about 6.6, thereby giving the intracellular fluids a positive charge.

With the extracellular fluid negative and the intracellular fluid positive, the potential difference or voltage built up is about *70 millivolts*. This is enough to exert a pull at each end of the charged rosette of proteins that is blocking the channel, causing it to stretch and thereby to open up the channel. Once this occurs, two things can happen. First, the upper negative end of the polar nutrients that are stacked on the outer membrane surface are attracted to the positive charge within the cell. Secondly, when 70 millivolts, created by the ionization of nutrients within the cell, causes the rosette to stretch and open, this upper negative end of the polar stack will be pulled towards the ion channel, which is now exposing the positive inner cell charge, causing the stacked nutrients to break off at some point and rush through the channels into the cell. Calcium can be the most effective such "*workhorse*", carrying up to *22 polar compounds*. Other cations carry much less; for example, potassium carries up to *only 8 polar compounds*. Both large ions such as potassium and smaller ions such as calcium are prevented, by the inward flowing nutrient radicals, from leaving the cell through the open nutrient channel. The second thing that occurs when the channels are sprung open by the voltage build up is that the smaller, positive cations within the cell, such as calcium and sodium, are attracted out of the cell by the negative extracellular fluids to which they are now exposed. These cations usually leave through specific, smaller ion channels that are also opened by voltage buildup. Now that the negatively buffered nutrients have entered the cell and the positive cations have left, the original conditions have been restored to a pH of 7.4 both inside and outside the cell. Thus, the cell wall has been depolarized, the calcium rosette is once again plugging the nutrient channel, the cell activity has been initiated, and the cycle is ready to repeat itself.

It should be noted that only some of the cations leave the cell. At a pH of 6.6, some of the calcium can bond to phosphate forming an almost insoluble calcium phosphate, apatite, which is thus secured within the cell to be stored for use when needed. It is also known that the extracellular fluid is lean in potassium while the intracellular fluid is rich in potassium. This is because of the potassium ion's large size which prevents it from leaving the cell through the small ion channels, while allowing it to readily enter the cell through the large rosette openings in the nutrient channels.

It should also be noted the voltage, or potential difference between the outer cell membrane and the inner cell, of 70 millivolts can be created whenever the internal ionization is greater than the external ionization, *regardless of pH*. The 70 millivolts is created in the healthy cell when the negative external pH is 7.4 and the internal pH is 6.6. When the cell is unhealthy with the external pH being positive, say in the positive 6.5 pH range, the 70 millivolts potential difference is created by internal positive cell ionization making the internal pH even more positive, say pH 6.2. Even lower pH's can also readily create the potential difference of 70 millivolts required to open the rosette nutrient channel. However, these acidic states tend to break down the cell membrane releasing the large ions, such as potassium, and strontium, thereby accelerating the acidification, or *self-digestion of the cell*.

Since the cells require combustion of food for energy, the first reaction that occurs is *glycolysis*, which is the *anaerobic* (absence of oxygen) breakdown of the body sugar glucose, by the reaction with adenosine triphosphate, ATP, which was produced from the photosynthesis of digested carbohydrates. In this reaction, two ATP molecules combine with one glucose molecule to create two more ATP molecules, lactic acid, and other by-products, while giving off energy in the form of heat. Then a series of chemical transformations, known as *the Krebs cycle*, occurs where the lactic acid and byproducts of the glycolysis are consumed, using *oxygen*, to produce nucleotide radicals, ATP and heat. A total of 36 ATP molecules are produced for each glucose molecule reacted. If enough oxygen is not present, the cell then uses glycolation to produce its required energy, resulting in the accumulation of lactic acid in the cell, which can eventually result in the death of the cell. However, calcium buffered mildly alkaline cellular fluids can provide adequate oxygen for the Krebs cycle to occur, thus preventing and/or reversing the buildup of the toxic lactic acid.

All of these explanations make calcium the key biological regulatory ion, regulating the pH and both the cell membrane's voltage and channel openings. It is also the key biological work-horse, bringing the most nutrients into the cell. Every child knows that milk (calcium) builds strong bones. With all four of these important biological functions being governed by calcium, it is important to thoroughly understand how calcium itself is regulated within the body. As has already been discussed, the entry of calcium into the body is regulated by the digestive process involving its ionization, other anions, and vitamin-D. But how is calcium cycled through the body?

Calcium is transported into the blood from the intestinal tract by way of specific calcium-binding proteins that are stimulated by vitamin-D. Once calcium is in the bloodstream, its deposition in bone is controlled by a hormone released by the parathyroid gland called *calcitonin*, which also, along with *inositol triphosphate*, controls both the removal and deposition of calcium in the cells. The parathyroid glands are regulated by the pituitary gland located directly behind the eyes as it is stimulated by *full spectrum sun-light* (Note: Glasses, especially tinted glasses, block much of the spectrum required for hormone regulation). Calcium resorption or removal from the bones is regulated by another hormone called the parathyroid hormone, which of course is also secreted by the para-thyroid glands. There are four pea size glands attached to the one ounce sized thyroid gland which is located around the larynx in the neck. When the amount of calcium deposited in the bones is the same as the amount removed, the system is balanced with no growth. However, when deposition is less, the bones become progressively weaker, *osteoporosis*, leading to numerous physical complications not only of the skeleton but of other organs and tissues as well. Thus it is important to understand what regulates the production of both of these hormones. Exposure to sunlight is the crucial factor.

As was discussed in **Chapter 6**, excess phosphorous in the digestive tract as may be caused by the over-consumption of red meat which has thirty parts of phosphorous for every one part of calcium, causes the calcium to *precipitate out* in the form of apatite, which *passes through the body unabsorbed*. Likewise, too much blood serum phosphorous with a deficiency of blood serum calcium, stimulates the parathyroid glands to produce larger amounts of the parathyroid hormones which results in the removal of calcium from the bones, raising the level of calcium in the blood. This is probably due to the need to maintain the calcium ortho-phosphate level in the serum and thereby maintain the critical pH of 7.4. Not surprisingly, higher levels of blood serum calcium stimulates the parathyroid glands to produce larger amounts of the calcitonin hormones which results in the deposition of calcium in the bones in the form of apatite. For obvious reasons, removal of the calcium from bones would be a last resort for the body; a robbery of Peter to pay Paul. Thus, brittle bones have a lot more to do with calcium deficiency than with old age.

The body's two kidneys, located behind the abdominal cavity just under the chest cage, also help to regulate the blood serum concentration of calcium. About *1700 quarts of blood flow daily through the kidneys* which filter materials from the blood, removing unwanted components as urine, while regulating resorption back into the blood all of the components necessary to sustain life. Thus, excess calcium is filtered out and passed out of the body through the urine while the balance is returned to the blood serum. It is also believed that some of the excess calcium can be stored in the kidneys for later use.

This brings us to the answer to the question of how stored calcium, in the cells, is released when needed. The answer is a special calcium releasing agent, inositol triphosphate. Inositol is a constituent of body tissue which is converted to the vitamin active triphosphate form, "INSP-3", *when stimulated with full spectrum light*. One function of this product of photosynthesis, INSP-3, is to increase the cationic permeability of the plasma membrane in the region of the cell that contains the photoreceptor, resulting in a flow of current to the cell that *stimulates specific glands to produce hormones*. The fact that inositol is absorbed from food sources such as vegetables, fruits, cereal grains, liver, kidney and heart, suggests that calcium storage plays a significant role in the function of these latter three organs.

At this point, it is essential to discuss the effects which certain other nutritious foods, that are not necessarily rich in calcium, can have on regulating the balance of calcium in the body. As was previously discussed, the consumption and digestion of food such as milk (*lactates*) and apples (*malates*) help by providing anions that help to keep the calcium ionized. However, foods that are mildly acidic, such as fruits and vegetables, possess another important capability. Once digested and absorbed by the body, their negative and mildly acidic anion radicals bond with the predominant positive and strongly alkaline cations, such as sodium and potassium already in the serum, resulting in *the formation of slightly alkaline and soluble salts* such as sodium lactate and potassium malate. Thus acidic fruits and vegetables (see Table #3) do not make the body fluids acidic. On the contrary, they help to maintain the critical and caustic serum pH of 7.4.

Mother Nature has chosen *"milk"* as its *ideal food* with which to begin life. Critics will state that humans are the only animals to continue drinking milk after breast feeding, and therefore continuing to drink milk is abnormal. Even the calves drink the cows milk for only a few months. However, the calves, like most other animals, replace the calcium rich milk with other calcium rich nutrients, such as 40 pounds of grass daily. Humans could also stop drinking milk, as long as they replaced the milk by consuming large amounts of other calcium rich nutrients, such as 30 pounds of grass or 15 pounds of spinach daily, which of course humans can not do. Thus, reducing milk consumption over the years can result in calcium deficiency induced diseases.

Unfortunately, a third of the aging population will develop osteoporosis which is a disease characterized by loss of calcium in the bones. This may be caused in part because of the lack of milk in the diet due to preference or due to intolerance to the lactose sugar component in the milk. This phenomenon probably occurs because the body is rejecting a nutrient that contains a substance it already has in excess. Lactose will produce lactic acid once digested. Lactose intolerant individuals may already have an excess of lactic acid in the cells that was produced as a result of cellular calcium deficiency dropping the pH of the cellular fluid below 6.5 and inducing the fermentation of glucose. Each glucose molecule produces, by fermentation, two lactic acid molecules. This lactic acid production drops the pH of the cell even further, thus preventing the cell from producing the basic nutrient radicals required for DNA synthesis. As was discussed in **Chapter 5**, the cells are starving themselves from both the life sustaining nutrients and oxygen. The body thus will reject milk to prevent further deterioration. Ironically, the body is suffering from severe calcium deficiency and desperately requires another source of calcium other than *its last resort, the bones*. Calcium supplements are the obvious answer to this dilemma.

For similar reasons, the calcium deposits in the tissues and joints of older people is also a sign of the calcium regulatory system adjusting to a severe calcium deficiency. The bony deposits reduce movement and cause pain and thereby limit activity in order to bolster the sagging skeletal structural strength resulting from the osteoporosis or decalcification of the bones. These *calcium deposits* which are a *direct result of calcium deficiency*, ironically enhance the fear of increasing calcium consumption, which would alleviate and correct the problem. Thus, some of the many diseases that are related to the last resort removal of calcium from the bones are osteoporosis, arthritis, rheumatism, sclerosis, and periodontal disease. Alzheimer's disease has been associated with aluminum accumulation in the body which in turn is associated with the overproduction of parathyroid hormones that stimulate removal of calcium from the bones. The source of the excess aluminum may be aluminum cookware, aluminum antiperspirants, aluminum based antacids, and unknowingly, *cheese burgers* because aluminum is added to the cheese to give it better flow properties when heated. It is interesting to note that for all of these diseases that are related to aging, many of their symptoms can be rectified by balancing the calcium regulatory system, a process perfected by Dr. Reich that will be discussed in another chapter.

A new study published by the University of Chicago in the January 2000 issue of *Cell* describes calcium's crucial participation in allowing the skin to keep fluids and foreign elements out. Dr Valeri Vasioukhin determined that "low calcium levels inhibit cell adhesion while high calcium levels promote it". She states that "As calcium levels increase, the puncta of adjoining cells forms into two rows, creating what researchers termed as an 'adhesion zipper'. When an adherence junction starts to form, the zipper closes to form a continuous sealed barrier between cells". She noted that "As calcium levels increased, projections known as filopodia extended out toward and entered neighboring cells binding them further". Thus calcium is a crucial component in holding the skin together.

Lastly, a discussion of the effects of one of Mother Nature's most nutritious foods on the calcium regulatory system is in order. *This food is sunlight!* It should also be noted that light entering the eyes influences the master glands, the pituitary and pineal glands, which control the entire endocrine system, including the calcium regulating parathyroid glands. The science of *photobiology* is a recent one. Light is definitely a nutrient essential to life and the triggering of hormones. Unfortunately, advances in technology have encouraged the past three or four generations of man to be the first to spend over half their lives under artificial lighting, which differs greatly from the full spectrum lighting like the sun. When "*artificial full spectrum*" lighting is used, human calcium absorption increases, *plants flourish and cows produce 15% more milk*. Full spectrum lighting is used to treat psoriasis, neonatal jaundice and herpes simplex infections. Tinted glasses can eliminate a large percentage of the sun's spectrum and therefore affect you both physically and psychologically. Thus, full spectrum light plays a vital role in the maintenance of a balanced hormonal system, and is therefore indispensable in maintaining a balanced calcium serum. It therefore appears that the calcium cycle that regulates good health can be summed up using Grandma's recipe, "*sunshine, fresh air, good food.*"

CHAPTER EIGHT

CALCIUM AND CANCER

A direct cause and effect relationship between calcium and disease was established in previous chapters. Could a similar relationship exist between calcium and cancer? The cancer experts say that there are too many types of cancer for there to be any possible common denominator, and yet these same experts would be shocked in disbelief by the demonstrable relationship between calcium deficiency and the diseases of aging, allergy and stress. There is also a great deal of evidence to show that calcium disorders play a pivotal role in diseases of the young, such as Duchenenne's muscular dystrophy, named for the lack of dystrophin protein in the cells. With muscular dystrophy, both the calcium channels of the cells are open much more of the time, and the calcium ion concentration within the cells is twice as high as normal. This indicates a calcium regulation problem. Also, allergies have been successfully treated as calcium disorders. With all of this myriad of human ailments related to calcium disorders, it would seem almost negligent not to discuss the probable integral role that calcium would play in the dreaded disease, *cancer*.

The definition of "cancer" according to the dictionary is "*a malignant tumor eating the part it is in, spreading indefinitely and tending to recur when removed*". In more technical terms *cancer arises when the deoxyribonucleic acid, DNA, is chemically altered, producing mutant cells that multiply without restraint and that produce a family of descendant cells that invade the surrounding tissues, with progressive emaciation.* This local invasion can be followed by metastasis, or spread to distant sights by way of lymphatics and the bloodstream, usually making cancer quite lethal. Some cancers can be killed by the use of chemicals (*chemotherapy*), by radiation, or by surgically cutting it out where possible, thereby destroying it *along with the part of the body* in which it resides,. Surgery usually leads over time to the spread of (the cancer into other parts of the body (*metastisization*). All must agree that the orthodox approaches are not satisfactory.

As the number of people being saved is growing, so too is the number of people dying from this dreaded disease. Billions of dollars are being spent annually on the search for the *"silver bullet"*, *a drug*, that will destroy the cancer without killing the patient. But, this is in contradiction to the orthodox stance that there is no one common denominator in cancer for the bullet to be shot at, especially since so many factors have been shown to trigger so many different types of cancer. Despite this, two time Nobel Prize Winner for Medicine, Otto Warburg, believed that the cause of cancer had been well defined which meant that there indeed could be a silver bullet, which he believed would be a combination of nutrients. If the silver bullet is to become a reality, a better understanding of the basic chemistry of cancer would be the best course in leading to the potential common denominator.

Everyone, including the American Cancer Society, agrees that there is a direct relationship between the occurrence of cancer and the foods we eat and the air to which we are exposed. But, that is analogous to saying that life causes death. What is really meant is that there are certain chemicals called *"carcinogens"* that are known to cause cancer when they are exposed in the body under specific conditions. For example, the existence of massive amounts of carcinogens by their sheer numbers can trigger cancer. Or, the addition of a third component, such as specific ultra violet radiation, can trigger cancer. In order to understand the existence of a common denominator, it would first be necessary to more thoroughly understand both the chemical nature of the carcinogens and the chemistry of their entry into the DNA template or mold.

Cancer was named by the ancients, after the great veins that usually surround the malignant growth, who compared them to the "*claws of a crab*" or "*cancer*" (Latin). Its origin was unknown and it was generally treated unsuccessfully with special potions, and on occasion, with local surgery.

By the turn of the twentieth century, orthodox medicine believed that cancer was *caused by* a variety of factors such as *"irritating substances, external injuries, the abuse of stimulating potions, immoderate indulgence in venery (sexual intercourse), the depressing influence of moral afflictions, bad food combined with the debilitating effects of cold and otherwise unhealthy habitations, and the injurious influence of one or more of these causes on particular organs"*. Also, *"the frequent occurrence of cancer in individuals for whom none of these predisposing causes seem to have cooperated in the production of the disease has led many pathologists to believe it as having an hereditary origin, the germ of the disease, or cancerous virus being transmitted from the parent to his offspring"*. Remedies at this time included local bleeding (which could reduce the tumor to 1/4 of its original size) by means of leeches, local compression, application of mercury or various preparations of iodine, and the removal of new growths by knife or by *their destruction by caustic applications*. At this time in history, the use of caustics was proven to have provided a *"permanent cure"* in many cases. (**Health and Longetivity**, Joeseph G. Richardsom, M.D., University of Pennsylvania. 1909, page378). Also note-worthy was the use of caustics with potassium iodide to successfully treat rheumatism.

By the 1950's, with cancer striking one out of every four people in North America, *the alkali treatments had long since been forgotten* and radiation was beginning to be used to kill the cancer and, unfortunately, surrounding healthy tissue. By the 1980's, with the incidence of cancer increasing, striking one out of every three people (see Table #6: US Cancer Deaths), chemical therapies (chemotherapies) were being perfected. Today, although there are many survivors, the incidence of cancer is still gaining in momentum and the *orthodox traditions and treatments*, which are obviously *loosing the war against cancer*, are firmly entrenched. We are only winning some minor battles. In order to change the course of history, we must gain a more thorough understanding of the chemistry of carcinogens and how they are energized to interact chemically with DNA, incorporating the electron physics involved in the cell membrane.

Table #6:
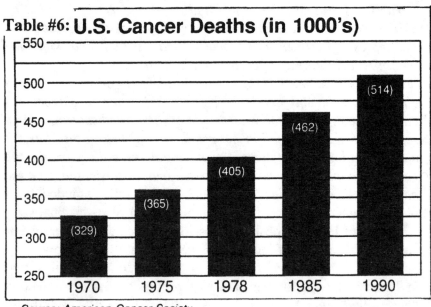

U.S. Cancer Deaths (in 1000's)

Source: American Cancer Society

62

All *carcinogens* are highly electrophilic (*electron loving*) reactants, or compounds that are able to produce electrophilic reactants within the body. These are free radicals, powerful electron acceptors, eager to gain electrons, that can enter the body through consumption of unsaturated oils, food additives such as nitrites, or through inhalation and skin absorption of toxic chemicals such as benzene and the tar of cigarette smoke. Most polycyclic compounds, or compounds with benzene rings and polar radicals, are carcinogenic. Once in the blood serum they aggressively react with strong electron donors such as *phosphorus oxygen bonding of the phospholipid cell membrane surface*. The bonding is strong, and the carcinogens therefore remain firmly attached to the outer surface of the cell membrane severely reducing the ability of the cell surface to polar stack nutrients for entry into the cell. If the cell membrane surface becomes significantly covered with the carcinogens, smothering the cell from its nutrients, the cell may begin to disintegrate, permitting entry of the carcinogen into the cell, thus exposing the DNA within the cell to the carcinogens.

It should be noted that carcinogens on the cell surface do not totally prevent nutrient stacking, since they usually do not cover the entire surface, and since the carcinogens polar radical is itself capable of doing some stacking. The danger with this latter prospect is that should the bond between the phospholipid cell membrane surface and the carcinogen weaken, due to excess electrons satisfying the positive charge of the carcinogen, the carcinogen could be ripped off the cell surface and follow the polar stack of nutrients, to which it is attached, into the cell, thereby exposing the DNA to the carcinogen. It is interesting to note that should the polar bond of the carcinogen on the cell membrane surface come in contact with a multivalent cation, such as *gold or platinum*, its electrical charge would be totally satisfied, thereby eliminating any participation in the stacking of nutrients.

Hence, unorthodox gold and platinum cancer treatments may indeed *have scientific merit.*

The weakening or breaking of the cell membrane to carcinogenic bonding could be the result of an "*excitonic*" process where exposure of the molecules of carcinogenic matter to radiation can cause two or more *electron couplets* to collide and undergo fusion, resulting in the liberation of electrons. An exiton is an electron couplet or triplet along with the positively charged hole that is created by the departure of the electrons from their normal orbital. The couplet exiton has two electrons, each spinning in opposite directions (this eliminates the production of a magnetic field), but moving together as a pair dragging their positively charged hole throughout the molecule. The triplet exiton has three electrons, two spinning in the same direction and one spinning in the opposite direction. This creates a magnetic field. Exiton fusion is the same process by which plants seemingly produce mass with less energy than can be calculated from the sun's photons. They photosynthetically produce glucose from carbon dioxide and water with seemingly less energy than is calculated as necessary, a process considered to be one of the *great secrets of life.* In this instance the small photon energy of sunlight energized exitons in the chlorophyll molecules to provide the required electrons (*energy*). Similarly, the electrons produced exitonically from specific radiation such as x-rays or nuclear radiation, stimulating the exitonically structured carcinogens, renders the previously positively charged carcinogens electrically negative, causing them to detach and repel from the negative phospholipd cell membrane surface, thereby liberating them for entry into the cell, where they can combine with toxic enzymes to form molecules capable of entering and mutating the DNA (*cancer*), to be discussed in detail later in this chapter.

The cell membrane can also begin to disintegrate due to the many processes of aging, some of which are the direct result of calcium deficiency producing low pH cellular fluids and causing *acidic self digestion*, as has been previously discussed.

Before explaining the carcinogenic alteration of DNA, a brief discussion of the *human genetic code* is warranted. To begin with, the human body holds about *ten trillion cells*. Large molecules called proteins determine the structure and function of each cell. A cell nucleus contains *twenty-three pairs* of *"chromosomes"*, that control the manufacture of proteins by the cell. A chromosome consists of *two* very long, spirally twisted *strands of DNA*, the chemical that carries genetic information from parents to offspring. DNA is divided into about *one hundred thousand clusters* called *"genes"*. A gene determines a human characteristic such as height, eye color, or disease resistance. Genes are composed of *thousands* of *"nucleotides"*, the smallest genetic unit. Nucleotides come in *four different shapes* called *"adenine, cytosine, guanine, and thiamine"* or "A, C, G and T" respectively, all arranged in pairs along the spiral strands of DNA. About *three billion nucleotides* make up the *human genome*, the blueprint of a human being, and man has only begun to chemically map their significance in the makeup of genes.

Exposure, alone, of the DNA to the carcinogens would be insufficient to create a mutation. Indeed, the body is believed to have several defensive mechanisms to fight off the invasion of carcinogens within the cell. For example, DNA is only able to accept certain specific radicals, and *the carcinogen by itself would not fit into the DNA strand*. Researchers, such as Dr. James P. Whitlock Jr., of Stanford University, know that carcinogens, such as *dioxin*, can bind with certain soluble intracellular receptors, toxic enzymes, to provide a new complex of *the right shape and size to be capable of binding to specific sequences of nucleotides, causing the DNA template to be bent or angled.* Once so altered, the DNA is capable of incorporating a foreign protein molecule that is not in the genetic code, in place of one of the A, C, G, or T nucleotides. Thus, a *mutant* may be born.

The question therefore arises as to what conditions within the cell are necessary to produce this mutation receptor ? The early work of Nobel Prize winner Otto Warburg, some seventy-five years ago, (*Cause and prevention of Cancer*; Biochem, Zeits, 152: 514-520, 1924), showed clearly that cancer was associated with *anaerobic (deficiency of oxygen) conditions,* resulting in fermen-tation and a marked drop in the pH of the cell (*Low pH Hyperthermia Cancer Therapy*; Cancer Chemotherapy Pharmo-cology 4; 137-145, 1980). Moreover, the production of mutation receptors cannot occur with the pH of the cell in the healthy calcium buffered 7.4 to 6.6 range, a range which assures the breakdown of glucose into the A, C, G and T nucleotide radicals that promote healthy DNA synthesis. M. Von Arenne showed that both high and low pH solutions *can quickly kill the cell.* He was also able to show that at a pH slightly above the normal pH of 7.4, the toxic enzymes which characterize the low pH cells are neutralized and that the cancer cells will enter a *dormant state.* Thus the success of the "*caustic solution treatment*" of tumors by the turn-of-the-century doctors could now be explained. Also, it should be noted that by definition, alkaline solutions are made up of hydroxyl (*oxygen-hydrogen*) radicals and therefore are oxygen rich. In the *absence of oxygen* within the acidic intracellular fluids, the *glucose undergoes fermentation into lactic acid,* causing the pH of the cell to drop even further, thereby *inhibiting the production of A, C, G and T nucleotides* that allow for normal DNA synthesis. This provides the necessary conditions for toxic enzymes to produce radicals that will bond with carcinogens. The complexes they produce will bind with specific sequences of nucleotides in the DNA, causing the template to be altered, thereby setting the scene for the abnormal replication of DNA to trigger cancer.

Thus, in the healthy, calcium buffered, slightly alkaline cell environment, *the conditions required for the propagation of cancer do not exist.* It therefore remains dormant, or dies. Dr. Reich noted that his cancer patients demonstrated: 1) lifestyle defects responsible for deficiency of one or both calcium and vitamin-D, 2) symptoms and physical signs of ionic calcium deficiency syndrome, and 3) a greater than normal incidence of these ionic calcium deficiency diseases. Thus, he considered cancer as the ultimate adaptation to ionic calcium deficiency, *"tailor made"* to survive and to thrive in an ionic calcium deficient environment. Dr. Reich found that the cancer in many of his patients seemed to go into remission once their calcium deficiency was rectified, by a change of lifestyle including diet and with mineral and vitamin supplements that raised the pH of their cellular fluids. Their associated ionic calcium deficiency diseases were also suppressed.

Another interesting fact is that cancer is virtually unknown to the **Hopi Indians** of Arizona and the **Hunza** of Northern Pakistan, so long as they stay in the same environment; this strongly suggests that something they are consuming is protecting them from cancer. The only significant difference is their water supply. The Hopi water is rich in *rubidium and potassium*, and the Hunza water is rich in *cesium and potassium*, making both of the water supplies rich with very *caustically active* metals. Researchers such as Dr. K. Brewer (*The Mechanisms of Carcenogenesis*, 1979, Journal of IAPM, Vol. V, No.2) and Dr. H. Sartori (*Cancer - ? Orwellian or Eutopian*, Life Science Universal Inc., 1985), found that, by not only addressing the calcium deficiency, but by also using these minerals to raise the pH to above the 7.4 range to a pH of 8.5, *the cancer cells would die while the healthy cells would thrive*; thus, once again verifying the observations of both the turn-of-the-century doctors and men like Dr. Reich. Both Brewer and Sartori would treat their cancer patients with the salts of both rubidium and cesium. These salts have large and extremely alkaline metal ions that can enter the cells through the large nutrient channels, but, like the large potassium ions, they have great difficulty in getting out of the cell due to the small ion cell exit channels. Thus, under these oxygen-rich, alkaline conditions, cancer cells die quickly, with no damage to the healthy cells, and therefore no serious side effects. The decomposing dead cells provide the nutrients for the renewed health and normal DNA replication. In his publication, *Cesium Therapy in Cancer Patients*, Sartori describes the two week treatment of 50 last stage, metastisized, terminal cancer patients (13 comatosed), with cesium chloride salts. Ten of the patients had breast cancer, nine had colon cancer, six had prostate cancer, four had pancreas cancer, five had lung cancer, three had liver cancer, three had lymphoma, one had Ewing sarcoma pelvis, one had adeno cancer, and eight had unknown primary cancer. With all fifty patients, conventional treatment had failed and the patients had been sent home to die. All were expected to die within weeks, with the survival rate being less than one in ten million. After 1 to 3 days, the pain disappeared in all of the patients. After 2 weeks, 13 died with autopsies showing no presence of cancer. After 12 months, 12 more had died, but 25, or *an astounding 50% survived*. Unfortunately, both cries of "*quackery*" and persecution from the medical establishment have driven this caustic cancer therapy research, started by Nobel Prize winner Dr. Otto Warburg, underground. (see web page www.cureamerica.net)

Dr. Max Gerson was world famous for *curing* supposed incurables, the most famous being *Albert Schweitzer* (**A Cancer Therapy: Results**, 5th Edition, Max Gerson, M.D., Del Mar, CA: Totality Book Publishers, 1958, 1975, 1977). Gerson often used **three caustic potassium salts** to successfully treat his cancer patients: potassium gluconate, acetate and phosphate. He knew that potassium was supposed to be a normal constituent of the cell serum, and should also be found in moderate amounts in blood serum. However, Gerson observed that many of his cancer patients showed *abnormally high levels of this mineral in blood serum.* To the horror of his medical colleagues, he fed these patients large doses of his potassium mixture in juices and found that the potassium level in their blood serum dropped very low as they made fast recoveries. The very alkaline potassium was going back into the cells where it belonged, raising the intracellular pH and thereby *inhibiting the proliferation of the cancer.* Gerson also found that an intravenous treatment of 90% oxygen and 10% ozone injected into the vein, with a very thin needle so that the bubbles of gas were tiny and the gas was quickly absorbed, would attack the malignant tissue on contact. Since the cancer cells are anaerobic, the addition of oxygen is incompatible with, and assists in reversing the production of toxic enzymes thereby disarming cancer's trigger mechanism

Other researchers have recently found that cancerous tumors cultured in a serum deficient in calcium, *will grow prolifically*, while the same tumor cultured in a serum rich in calcium *remains dormant.* They reason that calcium maintains cell adhesion and that this adhesion has a profound effect on the cancer, preventing it from spreading apart and breaking up. Furthermore, further research has shown that normal cells must be spread out on a solid substrate before they are able to initiate normal DNA synthesis, and that calcium is specifically required for spreading. This calcium induced cell spreading, while encouraging normal DNA synthesis, strongly inhibits abnormal syntheses (**The Role of Calcium in Biological Systems**, Volume 1, pages 157 and 169, CRC Press, 1985).

If all of this calcium is so good at inhibiting cancer, then why is *hypercalcemia* (high calcium in the blood) associated with various types of cancer? Hypercalcemia, which usually occurs in the latter stages of certain cancers with large tumors and metastasis, could be the body's last ditch defense mechanism. This defense is accompanied by *hypophosphatemia* (a low blood serum phosphate) and a *high calcium phosphate renal discharge*. The calcium within the cancerous and very acidic cells (pH as low as 4) will precipitate out as phosphate (Dr. Anghileri, **The Role of Calcium in Biological Systems**, Volume 1, page 46, CRC Press, 1985). To counter this loss in ionic calcium, the cancer cells obtain the calcium from other healthy nearby cells. But, as the cancer becomes massive or widespread, the calcium within is locked up in the phosphate form, and the most available source for the required calcium is the *calcium-rich bones*. When this happens, the blood serum becomes *very high in calcium* while the bones undergo *massive deterioration*. The blood serum is now high in calcium and low in phosphate, as much more phosphate is required for the *now dominant but less efficient sodium ion* to feed nutrients into the inside of the acidic cell, as was the case when the calcium was feeding nutrients into the alkaline cell. Under these conditions, the intestine finds it difficult to absorb digested calcium. The result is the whole calcium cycle system is now totally out of whack. Ironically, despite the very *high serum calcium*, what the system needs to put itself back into balance is more calcium from an external source, as well as sunshine and all of the other nutritious foods, in order to start the individual on the road to recovery. For these and other reasons, it can be demonstrated that many of the unorthodox cancer treatments *may indeed have scientific merit*, and that, when chemically understood, *cancer may be beaten painlessly*.

Thus the preventive medicine approach would be to replenish the depleting stock of ionic calcium through nutrition (see Table 3) and food supplements (see Table 8), thereby removing the need for the body to ravish calcium from the bones. On the other hand, the approach of orthodox medicine would be to find a *"drug"* to block the calcium from entering the cancerous cell, thereby *treating the effect but not the cause* of the problem, which is ionic calcium deficiency.

Coincidentally, orthodox cancer researchers "have recently recognized a new class of synthetic compounds called carboxyamide aminoimidazoles (**CAI's**) which, when administered orally (in animals) block the growth of established metastasis by altering the flow of *calcium* into cancer cells *(Cancer Cell Invasion and Metastasis,* Lance A. Liotta, **Scientific American,** February 1992)."* It may be that the CAI's reduce the level of the acidity which promotes both the solubility of bone mineral *(Calcium Homeostasis: Hypercalcemia and Hypocalcemia,* Dr. Gregory R. Mundy, University of Texas) and tumor calcification, as is also the case with the chemical ethanolamine, a very strong alkali which cancer researchers found to also reduce calcium hydrogen phosphate precipitation *(***The Role of Calcium in Biological Systems,** Volume 1, page 47, CRC Press, 1985). Likewise, nutritious alkaline foods (Table 3) also reduce the level of acidity, but without any toxicity or side effects. Such food also replenishes the dwindling supply of ionic calcium.

Other foods, such as polyunsaturated fats found in corn and other vegetable oils increase the formation of DNA-damaging free radicals (free radicals are "starved" for electrons and therefore thrive in mineral deficient acidic body fluids but are irradicated in mineral sufficient alkali body fluids). Women who eat five grams of these polyunsaturated fats daily *increased their breast-cancer risk by 69 per cent.* However, a study released in January 1998, led by Alicja Wolk at the Karolinska Institute in Sweden, which included the participation of the Harvard School of public health and was conducted on 61,471 women aged 40 through 76, found that the daily ingestion of at least 10 grams of monounsaturated fat (the kind found in olive and canola oils) - about three-fourths of a tablespoon - *cut the risk of breast cancer in half.* Another study released in November 1997 by the University of Maryland found that by taking huge doses of vitamins (20 times the RDAs of vitamins C and E) before consuming high fat foods like a cheeseburger of fries, the blood-thickening triglycerides are only

71

produced in small amounts. Also and the blood vessel expansion remained constant, thereby protecting the body from blood clotting and reducing the risk of heart disease. In addition, a December 1997 study by Matthew Gillman of the Harvard Medical School found that *"raising" the fat in the diet from 26 % to 35 % of total calories resulted in a 30 % reduction in ischemic strokes.*

Unfortunately, as is the case with most degenerative diseases, the orthodox choice is to employ noxious drugs to block the effect rather than nutritious food to cure the cause. Hippocrates, the father of medicine, made his choice clear; *"food is your best medicine and the best foods are the best medicines."* Hippocrates used garlic and onions to suppress cancerous tumors. It is interesting to note that in the *Journal of the National Cancer Institute,* 1989, both U.S. and Chinese scientists reported a study the more people ate garlic and onions, known to contain anti-bacterial, anti-fungal and anti-thrombotic (aggregations of blood platelets) agents, the less likely they were to develop stomach cancer which currently is the most common cause of death among cancer patients on a global scale.

It can therefore be demonstrated that, as has been shown with many other diseases, there is indeed a common denominator in all cancers; and as in other diseases *the silver bullet for the treatment of cancer* may turn out to be *"the calcium factor."*

CHAPTER NINE

CALCIUM AND HEART DISEASE

After all of the discussion in the previous chapters on the *king of the bioelements, calcium*, it will come as no surprise that calcium ions also dominate the health of the heart, with the *king of diseases being heart disease*. The link between these two kings is cell deterioration. Since the general health of the cell is regulated by calcium, any deficiency in calcium causes the cell function to become deregulated and thereby prone to deteriorate. In the heart and arteries this deterioration results in a chain sequence of events that has come to be known as heart disease.

Over one hundred years ago Sidney Ringer's article entitled *"A Future Contribution Regarding the Influence of Different Constituents of the Blood on the Contraction of the Heart"* was published in the **Journal of Physiology**. This work described the fundamental significance of the calcium ion to the maintenance of cardiac contractibility. Although an accidental finding, this work was the important base from which much of the focus on biological calcium originated.

As has been previously described in Chapter 5, because of calcium's most efficient ionization potential, *the heart's electrical muscle contractibility* has been proven by researchers to be due to *calcium ionization*. The most important aspect of heart disease is not a function of the chemistry of the heart muscle, but rather the chemistry of that which passes through it, the blood.

The heart is a hollow muscular organ that maintains the constant circulation of blood by contracting and dilating. When the circulation of blood through one of the coronary arteries (which nourish the heart muscle itself) is restricted or temporarily stopped by restriction and/or blood clotting caused by disease of the wall of this artery, a coronary thrombosis, which causes the death of the heart muscle supplied by the plugged artery, or what is commonly referred to as a *"heart attack"*, occurs. *Heart disease is the number one killer* in North America, with *cancer a close second*.

Heart disease refers to all irregular conditions of the heart, the most predominant of which is the heart attack. This condition usually follows *angina* (heart spasms) or heart pain caused by over-exertion of the heart muscle during which the ability of the diseased artery to supply the heart muscle with oxygen was exceeded. This situation is created by a thickening and hardening of the walls of the arteries which diminishes the size of the lumen or opening in the artery. This diseased state of the wall of the artery, known as arteriosclerosis, is usually caused by the gradual buildup of plaque on the walls of the arteries that has been related to several factors of which lack of exercise and faulty nutrition are the most important. Thus the wide variance in the incidence of heart attacks has been related to differences in *diet and culture*. Economic, occupational and social differences produce variance in stress, diet, exercise, exposure to sunshine and other critical factors that can be related to heart disease.

The obvious question is what is *"plaque"*? It turns out to be a composite of material that builds up over the years. It is composed of collagen, phospholipids, fibrin, triglycerides, mucopolysaccharides, cholesterol, heavy metals, proteins, muscle tissue and debris, *all bonded together with calcium*. This plaque only builds up in arteries that deliver the blood to the various parts of the body, but not in the much thinner walled veins that return the blood to the heart. If cholesterol is the cause of plaque buildup, as is suggested by the medical community, then why doesn't the same cholesterol in the same blood cause the plaque to build up in the veins ? Obviously, *cholesterol is not the cause of plaque buildup* and therefore, the doctors advice that the elderly reduce their cholesterol levels is ill-advised. In addition, the prescription of billions of dollars worth of needless cholesterol reducing drugs each year can only result in potential harm to the health of the public. Cholesterol levels can be lowered safely through balanced nutrition.

Both veins and arteries are lined with the same smooth internal layer that is in contact with the circulating blood. Unlike the vein, however, *the artery has an outer circling muscular layer* that allows for expansion and contraction to regulate the blood pressure maintaining a gradual delivery of blood to the organs as well as an equal distribution of blood nutrients to all parts of the body. As was described in the previous chapter on cancer, a calcium deficient acidic cellular medium can result in cell breakdown. When this inner coat of muscle of the artery breaks down, it is replaced with immobile collagen, probably to protect the artery from bursting, which would result in instantaneous death. This rigidity causes the previously flexible internal layer lining the artery that is in contact with the blood, and the sub-internal layer between it and the muscle coat, to become agitated and to undergo inflammatory degeneration leading to a rupture. The April 1997 issue of the *New England Journal of Medicine, Kilmer McCully* M.D. agrees with this concept by suggesting a radical *"new"* medical theory that *cholesterol* is not the primary *"cause"* of heart disease, but rather, *"inflammation of blood vessel walls is the primary cause* of heart attacks and strokes". The resulting debris, caused by the acidosis degeneration, along with fibrin phospholipids and collagen creates a patch to repair the break. This results in the formation of open negatively charged locations for the positive calcium in the serum to bind. Next, polar stacking, as described in the cell membrane mechanism, occurs; polar (electrically charged oppositely at each end of the molecule) fats begin to stack on the calcium, with cholesterol being only one of many.

At this point a discussion of cholesterol is warranted. It is both only a minor and last stage participant of a process that was instigated by the cellular breakdown of the arterial muscle. As such, deposition of cholesterol, probably to prevent leakage of the acid damaged artery, along with triglycerides and mucopoly-saccharides, is not the instigator of atherosclerosis, as popular misconception would lead you to believe, but only *part of the reparative process* that prevents the body from bleeding to death.

Doctors advise the public to reduce the cholesterol level in the blood by reducing the amount of cholesterol in the diet. Thus the public is warned to reduce the consumption of the two most nutritious foods known, *eggs and butter*, both of which are rich in vitamins, minerals and essential amino acids. However both also contain relatively high quantities of cholesterol. The egg, which contains about 300 milligrams of cholesterol (N.B.: the body manufactures up to *2,000 milligrams* of cholesterol per day) also is the body's main source of *acetylcholine*, an essential neuro-transmitter. Thus we are asked to avoid eggs and risk senility. To make matters worse, we have been asked to substitute cholesterol-rich butter with cholesterol-free margarine. The problem, however, is that margarine contains partially hydro-genated fats known as *"trans-fats"*, which actually *promote* increased blood LDL ("bad") cholesterol levels. Nutritionist

Margaret A. Flynn, at the University of Missouri, found in an experiment involving 71 faculty members, "basically it made no difference (to the blood cholesterol level) whether they ate margarine or butter." This was probably because, although the butter adds cholesterol to the blood, the *trans-fats* in the margarine induce the body to produce more LDL cholesterol which ends up in the blood. Biochemist Bruce J. Holub at the University of Guelph in Canada states: *"At the very least, one has to ask whether cholesterol-free claims should be allowed on high-trans products."* Thus it looks like grandma was right when she said, *"butter and eggs are good for you."*

Important facts about cholesterol are that it is *a vital component* of the body, it is found in every cell, it is a component of steroid hormones such as testosterone and estrogen it is used to conduct nerve impulses, and it is present in large quantities in the brain and bile. Additionally, cholesterol is one of the constituents of the skin that is *crucial to the production of sun-on-skin vitamin-D*. Finally, but not least important, about 80% of all body cholesterol is not ingested in the diets, but rather, *is manufactured by the body*.

In the blood serum, cholesterol is found *esterified* (made into an organic salt) with fatty acids as a lipid, or fatty acid ester. There are two types of these lipoproteins: high density lipoproteins (HDL) and low density lipoproteins (LDL). The HDL is the good cholesterol, as people who have high levels of it in their blood, actually have less risk of heart disease. When the LDL levels go up in the blood serum, no matter what the hereditary culture factors are, there is a proportional rise in heart disease. Researchers found that eating a diet of trans-fats increased the bad LDL cholesterol level in the blood, while reducing the good HDL cholesterol level (Ronald P. Minsink, Martin B. Katanm *New England Journal of Medicine*, August 1990). Other researchers found that feeding animals pure cholesterol *does not lead to increased heart disease* unless the cholesterol is heat damaged or oxidized. In the **Encyclo-**

pedia of Biochemistry, Dr. W. Hartroft states *"It still has not been shown that lowering the cholesterol in the blood (by 20%) will have any protective effect for the heart and vessels against the development of atheroma or hardening of the arteries, and the onset of serious complications"*. Since Dr. Hartroft made this statement, low cholesterol diets have been confirmed in dozens of carefully controlled experiments *not to reduce heart disease.* Thus, cholesterol is only poorly correlated to heart disease.

Then *why the popular misconception that cholesterol is bad for you?* The over simplified evidence to back this belief is that cholesterol is found in significant quantities in the arterial plaque. The reason for this has been previously explained as the result of polar stacking, with cholesterol participating as only ingredients of the final nails in the coffin. Since doctors do not really understand how this coffin of plaque is constructed, and the chronology of events in the creation of disease, and since they are pressed by reports of the calcium and cholesterol content of arterial plaque, the recommendation is to avoid the final outcome by avoiding the cholesterol nail. Thus the search for the vital medical factors that could lead to a medical breakthrough, *such as the prevention of calcium deficiency, is ignored or terminated.*

If this logic were to be applied to other diseased parts of the body, then calcium, which is found in excess in the cancerous tumors and in the brain plaque of Alzheimer's and Parkinson's diseases, should also be reduced or eliminated from the diet. But, for the reasons we have previously explained, this would be an equal *disaster to human health.* It should also be noted that Alzheimer's disease is associated with a calcium-aluminum build-up in cortical cerebral arteries, and Parkinson's is associated with a calcium-aluminum-silicon buildup in lenticular cerebral arteries, both of which are the direct result of negative cellular breakdown, or the creation of a negative field in the artery, due to acid buildup within the cell. This condition is then followed by the familiar positive calcium polar stacking mechanism over the open negative field. *Calcium did not cause the problem*, instead, had it been present in the correct amounts in the first place, it would have prevented cellular breakdown by creating the critical 7.4 pH buffered serum to allow proper brain cell function and repair. Correct cytoplasmic calcium concentrations could also have prevented the breakdown, polar stacking and resulting arterial plaque or *"sores"* in patients with hypertension (high blood pressure). The presence of calcium and cholesterol as pall bearers at the cell's funeral does not mean that they were the instigators in the death of the cell and the heart. Rather, the truth is that calcium is the life of the cell which can eliminate the buildup of the coffin of plaque and thereby render the cholesterol nail harmless to the heart.

Calcium ions also play a central role within the heart muscle itself, as the excitation-contraction coupling and relaxation is accompanied by a rapid redistribution of calcium. With a defective heart, *"as the calcium ion accumulation ability declines so does the ability to carry out contraction and relaxation."* (**The Role of Calcium in Biological Systems**, Volume 1, page 135, CRC Press, 1985).

The British Medical Research Council recently completed a *10-year study* that looked at the health of *5000 men* aged between 45 and 59. *Only 1 per cent* of those who regularly drank more than one-half liter (about one-half U.S. quart) of milk a day suffered heart attacks in the study period, against *10 per cent* of those who drank *no milk at all* (a *ten-fold* reduction). Also, drinking more than the one half of a liter further reduced the incidence of heart attack. Dr. Ann Fehily, one of the team of researchers, states that *"the association between milk drinking and lower heart attack risk was **absolutely clear**, and there was no significance about what type of milk: full, semi skimmed or full skimmed."* Thus, the essential ingredient was *calcium*. Also, a 25 year study ending in 1997 by the Finland National Public Health Institute on 4697 cancer-free women aged 15 to 90, concluded that there was *"an overwhelming association between the high consumption of milk and the prevention of breast cancer compared to other factors"*. What makes these studies tragic is that they meet all of the prerequisites for scientific authentication that is apparently required by the AMA. and yet both studies go unheeded, despite the fact that heeding them could potentially reduce the death rate of heart disease, by *ten-fold*, thereby saving millions of lives, as well as providing a means for women to prevent cancer. The fortunate drug companies, and the doctors of America, reap hundreds of billions of dollars per year because of this AMA indifference to using milk nutrition to prevent heart disease and also caustic nutrition to prevent cancer. This indifference is also paid for with human suffering as well as hundreds of thousands of lives each year.

Thus, as has been shown for cancer and other diseases (such as the allergic auto-immune stress diseases, and other diseases usually associated with aging) *heart disease*, which is the number one killer of man, is also *caused by cell deterioration* caused by calcium deficiency. The importance of calcium in the body is now an established and indisputable scientific fact. Calcium is the *biological* glue that holds our cells together and provides the crucial conditions for life to flourish. So, without waiting two decades for the medical profession to catch up, how can we use this knowledge today? Fortunately, Dr. Reich has laid the groundwork for easy clinical evaluations, and, using this *unified concept of disease*, has developed diagnostic techniques and time- tested, proven, mineral supplemented, nutritional remedies that are able to withstand the tests of international science.

CHAPTER TEN

CALCIUM AND CARL REICH

Dr. Carl Reich was a product of one of the most orthodox and rigid medical systems in the history of man, and yet, from day one, he was known as a medical maverick. There is an argument that innovators are not products of the system, but rather they are born into it. Either way, the result is the rare and therefore unusual man who is forced to challenge an existing system that is always based on self preservation. As President John Kennedy said, *"Some men see things as they are and ask why? Other men dream things that never were and ask why not ?"*

When Carl Reich was a young man, his Austrian immigrant father from Vienna died of cancer at the age of sixty-two. His father had always been a sickly man, plagued from childhood with constipation, obesity, and in his later years, with severe migraine. He had never exposed more than his face, hands and arms to sunshine. The most nutritious food he consumed was his annual two glasses of buttermilk. In short, Carl never knew his father to be truly healthy and without pain, and, partly by accident but mostly by design, he chose a lifestyle that would not lead him in his father's footsteps.

Of course everyone knew that biologically, sons are apt to follow in their parents' footsteps, but also it was beginning to be understood that good health was a function of the way you live. Carl resolved to follow the healthy trends of life; eating lots of the natural foods that his God had put before him, especially vegetables, fruits, and most important of all, the milk of life. He also reasoned at an early age that, like all of the animals, humans should share in experiencing the joy of sunshine and physical exercise. So, from an early age, as Carl would say, he *"took to the hills"*, hiking the mountains while stripped to the waist for most of the day.

In the late 1930's and 1940's, Carl Reich was a medical student pursuing post graduate work. During that period, the benefits and the toxicity of mega-vitamin supplements were being researched and debated. Carl Reich enjoyed personal health not known to his father, Carl knew it was due to his healthy lifestyle, and he was therefore indoctrinated to the belief that many *ailments should be prevented and not treated*. Lifestyle meant that he had exposed his body to certain dietary and environmental factors that promoted good health, while avoiding foods that inhibit good health. Carl wanted more definition of these factors.

Thus, it was not surprising to find Carl in his final post graduate year researching the injection of drugs, such as mecholyl and adrenaline, that stimulated either of *the two balancing divisions of the autonomic nervous system* that control the functions of all the organs of the body, such as lungs, heart, liver, spleen, stomach, pancreas, adrenals, kidneys, colon, intestines, sex glands and bladder. *One division, the sympathetic system*, is concerned with rapid adjustments in emergencies, whereas the *other division, the parasympathetic system* is chiefly concerned with digestion and repair of wear and tear of the body. For example, sympathetic impulses speed the heart and slow digestion, whereas parasympathetic impulses do just the opposite. Interplay between the two systems usually keeps the body processes at a controlled rate of activity, much like the gas and break pedals can be used to maintain the constant speed of a car going up and down hills.

The intravenously injected drugs that Carl researched in his post graduate studies had produced four widely different blood pressure responses that were attributed to various levels of stress. However, Carl suspected that these responses were probably *more attributable to various stages of mineral deficiencies* that were affecting the autonomic nervous system which regulates blood pressure. The autonomic nervous system sends out one set of impulses that causes the muscle coat of the blood vessels to constrict; the other, to dilate. Carl reasoned that since much disease was attributed to unbalanced excitation of organs by the nervous system, the identification of such imbalance in the non-diseased person could possibly be utilized to predict the occurrence of impending disease. He became determined to assess such imbalances by analyzing large numbers of patients for the different symptoms and physical changes that were known to be caused by each of the two different divisions of the autonomic nervous system.

Therefore, when Dr. Carl Reich began in earnest his medical practice in 1950, he began his assessment of imbalanced excitation of organs, but on clinical grounds only, assessing and recording and logging each patient's symptoms as they occurred either associated with autonomically excited disease or not associated with such disease.

A predominant symptom of the ill was anergy (the lack of energy). For over 60 years it had been well documented that the most energetic component of the human body, the heart, received its energy supply from *the calcium ion*. Dr. Reich, with his hundreds of *sick milkless patients* and the memory of his once-a-year-buttermilk father, knew that there was a correlation between their anergy ailments and the lack of foods in their diets that contain calcium and other specific nutrients.

During this research in practice, in one decisive week in 1954, Dr. Reich treated four of his patients, who he had studied and determined to be *calcium deficient*, with intravenous injections of calcium. He followed up with calcium gluconate and halibut liver oil (rich in vitamin-D) by mouth. These patients were experiencing chronic diarrhea, chronic asthma, constipation, leg cramps, rhinitis and nasal sinusitis. The results he obtained from this therapy, which provided a rapid resolution of these symptoms and diseases, convinced him that *ionic calcium* had relieved the smooth muscle and increased secretion of mucous in both the lung and intestine. He concluded that the severe lung and intestinal diseases which these patients experienced was not caused by an *"allergic reaction,"* but rather, they were caused by an *"ionic deficiency reaction."* He then treated a seven year old boy who had experienced chronic asthma since birth, with calcium, vitamin-A and vitamin-D capsules and was happily amazed to find that *the asthma was almost completely relieved "within three days,"* and never reoccurred as long as the child remained on the supplements.

At this time in medical history, as is much the case today stress such as infection, trauma, starvation, worry and overwork, was believed to trigger disease. It was thought that the exhaustion of the adrenal adaptive system, which produces life sustaining hormones to regulate our metabolism and muscular energy, resulted in a biological adjustment, that, when-ever taxed and exhausted, resulted in the creation of what is known as an *"adaptive disease."* However, Dr. Reich believed that the pattern emerging from his clinical studies confirmed that stress could not play a decisive role unless the adaptive system had already been previously compromised by chronic deficiency of specific nutrients, namely calcium and vitamin-D.

By 1958, after observing and treating thousands of patients, Dr. Reich definitely concluded that chronic disease such as asthma, ileitis and colitis were not the results of the direct effect of ionic calcium deficiency on the lung or intestinal tract. Instead, he concluded that *these diseases were the indirect result of deficiency* and represented the breakdown of autonomically excited adaptive function in an attempt to compensate for its deficient state. Thus, Dr. Reich believed that *deficiency of certain nutrients caused the organs to become more vulnerable to disease.* He began to look on cases of *angina* (heart pain to the chest caused by over-exertion of a diseased heart) as "*asthma of the coronaries*"; on hypertension (high blood pressure) as "*asthma of the systemic arteries*"; and on forms of ileitis and colitis (inflammation of the lower intestine and colon respectively) as "*asthma of the intestinal tract*," and to treat them with preparations containing calcium and vitamin-D, exactly as he had treated his first cases of bronchial asthma. Thus, Dr. Reich quickly became known to his peers as a *"medical maverick".* Although amused by this, he would have preferred *"medical quack".*

Dr. Reich began to categorize all diseases based on whether they were adaptive (organs adapt by taking on secondary role) or non-adaptive ionic calcium deficiency diseases. (See Table 7).

Table #7: Diseases

Adaptive and Non Adaptive Organ Response

Disease	Type	Organ	Function	
			Primary function of organ	Adaptive response of organ to a deficiency
Chronic asthma	Spastic tube & vessel	Bronchi	Respiration	Retention of CO_2 Lowering of pH
Hypertension	Spastic tube & vessel	Body arteries	Blood circulation	Kinetic energy to chem. change
Heart spasms	Spastic tube & vessel	Heart arteries	Heart circulation	Control cardiac & body funtions
Ileitis	Spastic tube & vessel	Ileum	Digestive	producing alkaline secretions
Peptic ulcers	Spastic tube & vessel	Stomach	Digestive	More HCl & systemic pH rise
Diabetes	Metabolic	Pancreas & cells	Metabolism of sugar	Producing acids to help ionization
Osteoporosis	Skeletal	Bones	Physical support	Calcium loss by hormone, enzyme
Rheumatoid Osteoporosis	Skeletal	Bones	Physical support	Calcium loss by hormone, enzyme
Cancer	Genetic	Cells	Variable functions	An adaptive mutant
Constipation	Spastic tube & vessel	Colon	Fecal storage	No adaptive response
Eneuesis	Spastic tube & vessel	Bladder	Urine storage	No adaptive response
Dysmennorhea	Spastic tube & vessel	Uterus	Reproduction	No adaptive response
Migraine	Spastic tube & vessel	Cerebral artery	Circulation	No adaptive response
Chronic myostis	Skeletal	Muscle	Motion	No adaptive response
Alzheminer's	Brain, nerve tissue	Cortical tissue	Mental function	No adaptive response
Parkinson's	Brain, nerve tissue	Lenticular	Coordination	No adaptive response
Lou Gherig's	Brain, nerve tissue	Nerves	Conduction of stimuli	No adaptive response
HIV, AIDS	Immune & secretory	Secretory tissue	Immunity & adaption	Immunity & adaption

NOTE: Table 7 provides an index of disease created by mal-adaption (where the organ responds by taking on a secondary function) to the calcium deficiency state, and non-adaptive where the organ is directly affected by the calcium deficiency.

Dr. Reich further antagonized his medical peers by treating these diseases, which he attributed to deficiency, not with dangerous drugs that frequently had serious side-effects, but with nutrient and vitamin supplements. Instead of embracing his concepts and clinical procedures that produced an army of healthy and happy patients, the medical elite decided to ostracize him and applied the label *"megavitamin"* to his therapy. They thereby *"implied danger"*, as *"mega"* means huge (in the millions), and everyone knows that anything in excess is bad for health, especially huge amounts of vitamins. But nothing could have been farther from the truth, as the name and the therapy were a mismatch. His dosages were indeed above the recommended dietary allowance, which he referred to as *"legislated deficiency"*, but were also *dramatically below* the minimal toxic dose.

If medical logic was applied fairly, and given the history of the drugs that most physicians have prescribed and administered over the last century, most doctors could technically be called killer-drug therapists. On the contrary, no one has ever died from vitamins and minerals *in the low amounts (milligrams or thousands of international units) prescribed by Dr. Reich*. However, it is true that vitamins, when taken in *"extremely"* large mega doses (usually given in amounts dramatically more than **10,000 times** *the Recommended daily Allowances, or RDAs* or as Dr. Reich would say, the *Recommended Death Allowance*) have been known to cause headaches, dryness of the mucous membranes, liver problems, and in a rare few cases, if taken for a very long time, death. But, the necessities of life, (i.e. sugar, salt, water) if taken in excess for a long time, can also cause medical problems leading to death, as with *mega amounts*, all nutrients are toxic.

When vitamins were first discovered to have such great health enhancing properties, of course everyone went overboard.

In the 1920's and 1930's, for example, physicians *commonly prescribed 500,000 or more International Units (I.U.) of vitamin-D* daily for diseases such as arthritis. To put this amount in quantitative perspective, it should be stated that 1 milligram (a grain of sugar weighs about 10 milligrams) of vitamin-D equals 40,000 I.U.'s and the 500,000 I.U. daily dose weighed only 12.5 milligrams (about as much as a single grain of sugar). Thus vitamins were known as "*micro nutrient*" as so very little was required to create dramatically beneficial results. Despite this, in 1929, investigations were begun to determine if massive doses may be toxic to any individual. The results of the study on over 773 human subjects and 64 dogs was published in 1937 (*Further Studies On Intoxification With Vitamin-D* by I.E. Streck, M.D., H. Deutch, A.B., C.I. Reed, Ph.D., and H.C. Struck, Ph.D. from the College of Medicine, University of Chicago), and *concluded* that "both human subjects and dogs generally survive the administration of 20,000 I.U.'s of vitamin-D per kilogram of body weight per day for indefinite periods *without intoxication.*" This means that a woman weighing 110 pounds could safely take 1,000,000 I.U. daily. The study, not surprisingly, found that massive doses, as high as 500,000 I.U. per kilogram per day, equivalent to 25,000,000 I.U. per day (*over 62,000 times the RDA*) for a woman weighing 110 lbs., might cause death. However, it also concluded that the cell injury and calcium deposition was "*both reversible and repairable* if administration is discontinued promptly." Finally, it concluded that "intoxication for short periods *does not result in any permanent injury.*" Ironically, further studies in the 1940's (*Comparative Therapeutic Value and Toxicity of Various Types of Vitamin-D*, by C. Reynolds, M.D., Louisiana State University) suggested that the toxicity of the massive doses given in this study, was probably due to the chemical impurities in the first vitamins manufactured (a problem that had been since corrected) rather than due to the vitamins themselves, and concluded that their findings were the same as Struck, that *vitamin-D was non toxic in amounts under 20,000 times the RDA.*

Despite the scientific evidence to the safety of vitamin-D when taken in the moderate amounts several times the RDA, which resulted in spectacular health benefits, the medical authorities, with no scientific support, *deemed* that any risk at all was unwarranted, and therefore they recommended the consumption of only minute quantities of any vitamin. Thus in the 1940's and 1950's the doctors began recommending that their patients consume only trace amounts of vitamins, 400 I.U. of vitamin-D for example. Ironically, when it came to making money for the drug companies, they routinely prescribed popular drugs such as *Dalsol, Deltalin and Drisdol, all of which contained 50,000 I.U. of vitamin-D*.

The party-line trace quantities that they were recommending to their patients *had been arbitrarily determined* by the medical authorities and had no scientific merit. In fact, Recommended Daily Allowances (RDAs) of vitamins and minerals were based on the amounts of these nutrients already present in what was considered to be the *typical American diet*, and even this approach was inaccurately assessed. For example, they recommended only *5,000 I.U.* (international units) *of vitamin-A daily*. To show how ridiculously low an intake 5,000 I.U. really is, a man eating a modest meal of carrots and liver consumes 100,000 I.U., and without a doctor's prescription! Spinach, sweet potatoes, red peppers and dried apricots would also be disallowed from the doctor's prescribed meal. Warnings are also given that "vitamin-A is poisonous, because *eating polar bear livers*, an especially rich source (over 8,000,000 I.U. of vitamin-A per pound), *can be fatal*", as was reported in February 1991, **Scientific American**, "*The A Team*" by T. Beardsley). Of course, eating *1600 times* the recommended daily dose *of anything*, including water, could be hazardous to your health. Contrary to some reports, the early explorers *did not die* from eating polar bear livers, but rather, they experienced exfoliative dermatitis and loss of hair. It is also interesting to note that in 1988, a Swedish team of scientists discovered that the polar bear and seal livers tended to accumulate cadmium metal contained in the polar waters. The symptoms for *cadmium poisoning* are exfoliative dermatitis and loss of hair. Vitamin-A has also been shown by several scientific studies to *inhibit cancer*; the amount necessary, however, is 20 times the recommended daily allowance (*Diet and Cancer*, Lenard A. Cohen, **Scientific American**, November 1987). Despite these scientific facts, most doctors remain erroneously convinced that vitamin-A in large amounts is toxic.

Other vitamins, such as vitamin-D, were also *considered to be dangerous*, except in exceedingly low dosage, by the medical authorities. Only 400 I.U. were allowed, this despite the fact that the human body can generate up to 163 I.U. for each square centimeter of skin (P.C. Beadle, **"Cholecalciferol Production"**) or 3,000,000 I.U. over a good sunny day at the beach. Also, only 1200 I.U. or 60 milligrams of vitamin-C are recommended; this despite the fact that you exceed your daily dose with the first glass of orange juice. Nobel Prize winner, Dr. Linus Pauling recommended up to 5000 milligrams (100,000 I.U.) daily, while Merv Griffin tells his audience that he takes 2,500 milligrams (50,000 I.U.) daily and has not had a cold for many years. Indeed, some of these latter amounts of vitamin-C may seem high; however, they have been tested by men of science who successfully practiced what they preached.

Despite this *logical scientific argument against the RDA's*, the Food and Drug Administration (FDA), the self proclaimed "protector" of health of Americans, expended considerable effort unsuccessfully in the early 1970's to make a drug prescription necessary, making it a *criminal offense to purchase vitamins and minerals* containing more than 1-1/2 times their RDA's. The resulting public outcry prevented the FDA from legislating RDA's poor health consequence.

$\textbf{D}$r. Reich recommended *very moderate doses*, only a small fraction of the so-called minimal toxic dose, of both vitamins and minerals for moderate amounts of time, in addition to a change in lifestyle, and then a substantial reduction once the desired results had been achieved. This was done while carefully monitoring the patient's blood, urine and medical symptoms. By 1972, he had added *the pH salivary test* to his health checks and found that this quick and inexpensive test provided immediate evidence of calcium deficiency (this will be discussed in detail in the next chapter). For a Schedule of dosages by Dr. Reich in three age categories, see Table 8.

TABLE 8: Schedule of Initial Dosages of Vitamins and Minerals
(These are maintained for several weeks or months and then reduced to one half to one third)

Patient (Age)	Vitamin-A (I.U.)	Vitamin-D (I.U.)	Calcium (milligrams)
3-6	5,000 to 8,000	1,000 to 2,400	250 to 500
15	30,000	4,800	750
Adult (160 lb)	54,000	7,200	1,250

Note: 1. Dosage given was average number that adjusted slightly up or down depending on weight.
  2. About half of the dosages of vitamin-A and vitamin-D was given in the form of Halibut liver oil, and half in water soluble form, "Aquasol A and D".

$\textbf{O}$ver the years, the patients that Dr. Reich had treated for *diseases attributed to calcium deficiency*, also developed resistance to chronic and recurrent infection as he corrected their calcium deficiency. As a result, beginning in 1983, one year after the new HIV viral disease had been described as *"acquired immune deficiency syndromes"* (AIDS), Dr. Reich suggested that this disease may represent both immune and *"adaptive"* deficiency. He therefore coined the acronym *"AAIDS"* to more

91

correctly describe the disease. Since only some of those who carry the virus develop the disease, the prior state of the individual's immune and adaptive defense systems must play a key role, and the calcium ionic factor is pivotal in the state of immunity. A calcium deficient asthmatic has a severely weakened defense against the cold virus; thus, calcium deficiency may also render an individual exposed to the HIV virus incapable of preventing the virus from *"getting a toe-hold."* This is in keeping with the discoveries which biochemists have recently made proving *ionic calcium to be a most vital factor in all biochemical mechanisms* responsible for cell function.

Later in 1983, with a flourishing practice in which he had treated up to twenty thousand patients without one complaint to the medical authorities, Dr. Reich was forced to follow in the footsteps of those famous medical innovators before him, to have his license to practice medicine canceled by an elite medical body, by the College of Physicians and Surgeons. His *"crime"* was that he was not following their medical guide lines with his simple and extremely effective medical concepts and practice. He was considered to be *"potentially dangerous"* to the patients. But, as you shall see from his record as a physician, he was more potentially dangerous to the other physicians, lest their patients finally discover the truth. For a list of Dr. Reich's patients categorized by disease, numbers of patients and medical successes, see Table 9.

From the very beginning of Dr. Reich's medical career, he had postulated reasons for the importance of calcium in human health. As he began to treat patients successfully in increasing numbers, his convictions grew even stronger, and he began to see even more connections between disease and calcium deficiency. This led him to postulate a *"Unified Concept of Disease"* involving *calcium deficiency*, which made him appear even more radical to his medical peers. Unfortunately, he was not aware of the truly massive amount of research being carried out on cellular calcium in the scientific community, giving credence to his postulations.

Table 9: Patients Treated with Vitamins and Minerals by Dr. Reich

Type of Disease	Number of Patients	Good to Excellent Resolution
Adult Chronic Asthma	5,000	67 %
Child Chronic Asthma	6,000	93 %
Rheumatoid Arthritis	100	60 %
Osteo Arthritis	2,000	60 %
Dermatitis & Rhinitis	1,000's (many)	NS
Bursitis & Rheumatism	1,000's (many)	NS
Anxiety & Depression	1,000's (many)	NS
Fatigue & Depression	1,000's	NS
Migraine	100's (many)	NS
Ileitis & Colitis	100's (many)	NS

Note: 1) Patients were not treated specifically for cancer.
2) NS - Means not surveyed.

Although the numbers of therapeutic successes in Table 9 look impressive, the real success is *the spoken word* of the thousands of patients who revere Dr. Carl Reich and are passionately grateful to him for succeeding where orthodox medicine had failed. But for Carl, his most successful patient was himself. He had led a productive and healthful life, with both sound mind and body, and had no intention of stopping. He had happily gulped down his once-a-day-milk and taken his dietary supplements allowing himself to enjoy healthy recreational activities in his 80's, while the *younger once-a-year-buttermilk ghost of his father* looked on with envy.

In the September/October 1996 issue of **City Scope**, a well read magazine in Calgary, Canada, the city where Dr. Carl Reich practiced medicine, a feature article "*Ahead of His Time*" was published as a tribute to his pioneering efforts with preventive medicine. The article refers to Dr. Reich as the "*Father of Preventive Medicine*", and gives him the main credit for having Bill 209, known as the Medical Profession Amendment Act, passed in the Province of Alberta Legislature. The bill simply states: "*a registered practitioner) shall not be found guilty of unbecoming conduct or found to be incapable or unfit to practice medicine or osteopathy solely on the basis that the registered (practitioner) employs a therapy that is non-traditional or departs from the prevailing medical practices, unless it can be demonstrated that the therapy has a safety risk for that patient unreasonable greater than the prevailing treatment*". Thus, for the first time in North America, a government has put the burden of medical proof on the accuser. Unfortunately, although Dr. Reich took pride in the bill's passage, he noted that "*these Doctors know what's in the best interest of their careers, even if it 's not in the best interest of their patients*". When Barefoot took Reich his first copy of the magazine, Reich responded that "*unfortunately, the article was written ten years too late for me because I'm getting too old to really take advantage of the new law*". Two months later, Dr. Carl Reich, the *Father of Preventive Medicine*, passed away in his sleep.

There is an argument that innovators are not products of the system, but rather innovators are born into the system. Either way, the result is the rare and unusual individual who is forced to challenge the existing system, which is always based on self preservation. If America hopes to turn the tide against disease, the dreamers must prevail, thus the following quote is worth repeating:

"*Some men see things as they are and ask why? Other men dream of things that never were and ask why not?*" (President John F. Kennedy).

94

CHAPTER ELEVEN

CALCIUM AND SALIVA pH

One of the most important developments in Dr. Reich's research on deficiency disease was the development of *a simple, yet accurate, clinical test for calcium deficiency.* When healthy, the pH of blood is 7.4, the pH of spinal fluid is 7.4, and the pH of saliva is 7.4. Thus, *the pH of the saliva parallels the extracellular fluid.* As we have seen discussed in previous chapters, the calcium (mono) orthophosphate is a major component of these chemical buffer body fluids that tries to maintain the pH at 7.4. We have also seen in previous chapters that this pH is critical in promoting both normal DNA synthesis, cell growth, cell function, and cell repair. As the level of the chemical buffer drops in these serums, so too does the ability to maintain this critical pH. *The calcium ion level therefore has a direct reflection on the pH.* This can be measured by a simple three second, two cent, pH test of the saliva that provides an immediate indication of the state of the calcium ion level, and thus indirectly *the state of our health.*

As has also been previously explained, the pH of the fluids inside the cell drops from the alkaline negative pH of 7.4 when the channels are open, to as low as the acidic positive pH of 6.6 (Table 2) after the channels close and the nutrients have been chemically altered and consumed by the cell. This change in pH creates the potential difference (*voltage*) between the inside cellular fluids and the outside fluids, resulting in the channels opening again. This process is repeated indefinitely like a cell "*breathing*" process. When discharged into the cell, this electrical potential activates all of the biological processes that are responsible for cell function and nerve stimulus. If the pH of the extracellular fluids falls to a level lower than 7.4, say to a pH of 6.5 *due to chronic calcium deficiency*, then the intracellular fluids must drop lower, to about 6.3, to produce the same electrical voltage difference. This causes the nutrient glucose to stop producing the A, C, G and T radicals required for normal DNA synthesis, and instead to produce lactic acid, which drops the pH even further. The result is a weakening of the cell function. If the extracellular pH drops even further, the intracellular pH drops correspondingly, and may result in the production of *toxic enzymes* as well as cellular breakdown. These events are reflected in terms of *disease, the aging process, and the production of cell mutations*.

Mother Nature tries to keep these events from readily occurring by providing us with a *second buffer mechanism*: a mixture of potassium dihydrogen phosphate and disodium hydrogen phosphate that can maintain the extracellular serum at a pH of 6.8. Unfortunately, in this case, the large potassium ion has great difficulty in leaving the cell once it is inside; however, this does tend to raise the pH slightly. Thus this secondary support buffer system is much more limited in its capability of keeping the pH from dropping.

It is therefore evident that this physical-chemical pH test of saliva represents *the most consistent and most definitive physical sign of the ionic calcium deficiency syndrome*. Dr. Reich

96

found acidic pH directly related to lifestyle defects that supported the calcium deficiency, and to all of the various stages of developing ionic calcium deficiency and diseases. He found that when the deficiency created by defects of lifestyle were corrected by diet and dietary supplements, the pH rose as the disease regressed. This made this simple test an excellent means of monitoring of the progress of the therapy. It also enabled Dr. Reich to assess the general state of health of his patients within seconds and to assess their proneness to develop symptoms and *disease caused by ionic calcium deficiency*.

The pH paper can be obtained by the general public at any scientific supply company, (Micro Essential Labs, **718-338-3618**, catalog # 434), or through most pharmacists. It comes in various ranges, and the **range between 4.5 and 7.5** is best. The pH range of the non-deficient and *healthy* person is in the *7.5 (dark blue)* to 7.0 (blue) slightly alkaline range. The range from 6.5 (blue-green) which is weakly acidic to 4.5 (light yellow) which is strongly acidic represents states from mildly deficient to strongly deficient, respectively. Most children are *dark blue*, a pH of 7.5. Over half of adults are green-yellow, a pH of 6.5 or lower, reflecting the calcium deficiency of aging and lifestyle defects. *Terminal cancer patients are usually a bright yellow, a pH of 4.5*. This is over *1000 times* the acidity level of a normal healthy individual at pH 7.5, causing the body to self-digest. Also, acidic pH is exhibited by anxious and depressed adults, hyperactive children, and rebellious or delinquent adolescents. Psychologically, when a child sees that he is green, he will do almost anything to be "*blue like his buddies*", especially if they watched him being tested. The same is true for adults, especially when the test has any yellow. This test is extremely believable, as it provides demonstrable proof of biophysical change.

The test, although generally reflective of the state of health of the patient, may not always be accurate. For example, while it is easier to test the pH of saliva than the pH of the blood, due to the ease of acquiring a sample, the saliva pH could be influenced by some recently consumed food, thereby producing a false positive test. This can be overcome by *waiting for two hours* after putting anything in the mouth before taking the test. The patient should *also draw fresh saliva into his mouth and swallow it*, several times before taking the test. Also, because of a temporary aberration in the body, such as an adjustment for an over-consumption of some foods high in some contributing component such as phosphates or alcohol, the pH could be temporarily affected. Thus, *an acidic test should be re-tested two hours later* (See Table #12, page 119 for the Supplement Program)

If still acidic, a good nutritional practice would be *to adopt the mineral and vitamin therapy* as is described in Chapter 14: Recipes For Good Health, and as has been described in the previous chapter. This should also be augmented by *a change in lifestyle*: more oxygen intake (exercise) and exposure to full spectrum lighting (not necessarily sunbathing), accompanied by a change in diet to more fruits, vegetables, milk, eggs, butter, fish, and juices, with moderation in red meats (rich in phosphates) and alcohol. Avoid soft drinks, and in general, choose the foods you know are nutritious, remembering that anything, no matter how good it is supposed to be, is bad for you in excess (even too much water can kill you). And, above all, take it easy and relax, as you are embarking on a course of action that can set your biological clock back a few notches, allowing you to lead *a more healthy and productive life*.

CHAPTER TWELVE

CALCIUM AND ELECTROMAGNETISM

No discussion about the importance of any bioelement would be complete without a discussion about *the total environment in which the body's many biochemical reactions take place*, and not just the chemical environment. For example, it is well known that pressure and temperature, two physical parameters, can affect the outcome of many chemical reactions. Heat applied to acids dramatically speeds up digestion, while a vacuum applied to a liquid speeds up the chemical production of gases. Both pressure and temperature effects have been documented for hundreds of years. What has not been either documented nor understood by many is *the effects that electromagnetic fields have on biochemical reactions*.

What we have discussed in the previous chapters at some length are the bioelectrical fields that are created to open and close ion channels, or send electrical impulse signals to muscles, and give rise to secretion and motion. What has not been discussed is the fact that associated *with every electrical field*, according to the laws of physics, *is a propagated magnetic field*. Changing the intensity of the electrical field causes a corresponding change in the magnetic field. Likewise, when the magnetic field changes due to any external forces such as the overlapping of another magnetic field, there is a corresponding change in the electrical field. Thus, there would also be an *associated effect on the electro- bio-chemical reactions*, which could change the functioning of the human cell. This can be used beneficially to assist in the regulation of these electro-biochemical reactions.

One example of the associated effect on the body's electro-biochemical reactions is the use of *magnetic beds.* The pH of the saliva becomes alkaline after a few hours of body exposure on the magnetic bed. The magnetic field *induces the bicarbonate bonding to bend and break producing hydroxides*, thereby creating a negative, or alkaline pH extracellular fluid (see Table 10). The *benefits of this are twofold*, first the alkaline fluid by definition is physically capable of absorbing far more oxygen than the low pH positive fluid, and secondly, raising the pH of the external cellular fluid also raises the potential difference between the external and internal fluids thus allowing the nutrient channel to open more readily. This latter occurrence allows the cells to function in their more normal alkaline range. The increased oxygen along with the nutritional stimulus has a temporary but healthy purging effect on the body.

Exposure to uncontrolled magnetic fields can have just the opposite effect on the bioelectric body. This is a very scary proposition, as we live in an electrical world with pulsed electro-magnetic fields superimposed on us from all directions. In order to begin to understand the consequences, let us first turn the clock back in time to when humans were *basically free* from this electricity phenomenon.

We do not have to go very far, just a little over one hundred years to a time when our biochemical reactions were functioning free of external magnetic or electrical imbalances, just

Table 10: Magnetically Induced Chemical Reaction in Fluid

$$Ca(HCO_3)_2 \xrightarrow[\text{Field}]{\text{Magnetic}} Ca(OH)_2 \quad 2CO_2$$

Calcium bicarbonate   Calcium hydroxide   Carbon dioxide

$$pH\ 7.5 \xrightarrow[\text{Field}]{\text{Magnetic}} pH\ 9.2 \qquad \textbf{Water}$$

$$pH\ 7.2 \xrightarrow[\text{Field}]{\text{Magnetic}} pH\ 7.5 \qquad \textbf{Blood}$$

$$pH\ 6.2 \xrightarrow[\text{Field}]{\text{Magnetic}} pH\ 7.4 \qquad \textbf{Cellular Fluid}$$

STRUCTURAL CHARGE ORIENTATED REPRESENTATION

Molecular orientation without magnetic field	Molecular orientation with magnetic field	Reorganization of molecular bonding

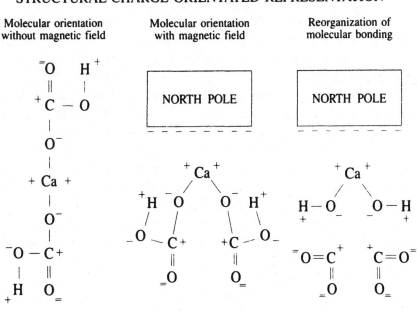

Calcium bicarbonate normal straight chain form	Negative magnetic field reorganizes structure of calcium bicarbonate	Calcium bicarbonate breaks into calcium hydroxide and carbon dioxide

as they had been evolving since the beginning of man. At that time, they were *balanced with nature*, especially sunshine and fresh air, and the earth's magnetic field, as man was just beginning the industrial revolution that was about to pollute the world. Electricity meant free work, and man was more than eager to happily smother himself in the explosion of new electrical gadgets, neither knowing or caring about the biological consequences.

Today, man is aware of both the air and water pollution, and is quite aware of the negative effects they both have on his body. However, most, if not all of the current establishment is *totally blind to the negative effects of "electro-pollution"* on the biochemical reactions going on in the human cell. This despite the fact that we all fear the effects of high frequency radiation such as x-rays and gamma radiation.

This is not to say that there are not some men who are extremely knowledgeable about electro-pollution, as indeed there are such men. Pioneers of electro-biochemistry, electrophysiologists, such as Dr. Robert Becker, who began his studies of regeneration (*re-growing of parts of the body that have been destroyed*) about the same time as Dr. Reich began his clinical research on calcium deficiency, knew from the very beginning that biochemical changes were related to orderly electrical events in the body. At that time, a stream of electrons had been measured flowing from the new wounds of both plants and animals. This *"current of injury"* could be correlated to reparative growth. In addition, the current of injury was proportional to the extent of the injury. Not since the dedicated physician Galvani had made a frog's leg twitch in 1791 with an external electrical source and then in 1794 made a frog's leg twitch by touching it to the dissected out (wound) spinal cord of the same frog, had bioelectrical currents of wounds been so graphically demonstrated.

Becker and the other pioneers found that *the regeneration of amputated limbs was proportional to the current of injury*, and began immediately to experiment to encourage regrowth with electrical stimulation (**The Body Electric**, 1985, Morrow, New York). Despite results that technically could be classed as exciting, research funds were cut off and huge establishment roadblocks were put in the way of further research. Both the regulatory medical elite and orthodox biologists did not like the concept that something that they knew so very little about could have such major consequences on something about which they were supposed to be the world authorities.

Also, another major biological event went ignored by most of the medical community. In the early 1970's, the surgeon Cynthia Illingworth of the Sheffield Children's Hospital in England accidentally found that when a young child's finger is sheared off beyond the outermost crease of the outermost or last joint, and the wound is dressed but not closed, *the finger will grow back* perfectly within three months. By 1974 Illingworth documented several hundred regrowth fingertips. Other pediatric surgeons, like Dr. Michael Bleicher of New York's Mount Sinai Hospital, have become confident of the infallibility of the process. Yet few hospitals accept this natural replacement procedure, as it has not been endorsed by the medical cartel, who are not swayed by visible facts that they do not understand. Further research in this medically forbidden field, as Dr Becker explains in his book **The Body Electric**, will one day lead to the *"regrowth of other human limbs"*, such as arms and legs.

It was known that *space flight osteoporosis*, decalcification of up to 8 per cent of the bones which occurs after only a few weeks in orbit, was probably *due to the unnatural electrical currents induced in the body*. These were produced by the rapid motion through the Earth's magnetic field, with polarity reversal every half hour resulting in induced biochemical cellular reactions. It was also known that cell division cycle time, which involves the duplication of all the cells' DNA and the chromosomes that are then distributed equally between two cells, *takes exactly one day.* This implies that tissue repair, that depends on regulated cell division, is synchronized with the earth's magnetic field. In the 1960's scientists overcame space osteoporosis by strapping on electromagnetic coils that approximated the bones' normal gravity stress signals, and stimulated cell growth by using pulsed electromagnetic fields at the Schumann rate of resonance that induced currents within the body from outside the body. In 1979, pulsed electromagnetic fields had been demonstrated as so effective in stimulated bone healing, that the authorities yielded to pressure and gave their rare approval.

Humans, therefore, naturally are *cyclic creatures* and the frequencies of magnetic radiation, measured in cycles per second or hertz and not just their intensity, become the over-riding parameter affecting bioelectrical responses. Electro-biologists have determined these interfering frequencies most detrimental to cellular bioelectrical functions to be between 1 to 100 hertz. This is in the extremely low frequency range (ELF from 0.1 to 100 hertz). Unfortunately, man chose to oscillate his electrical power supply *in the middle of the ELF range at 60 hertz.*

Many key bioelectrical reactions, such as the healing of wounds, are controlled by electrical potential differences as little as 0.00006 volts. Exposure to radio waves at 16 hertz *dramatically increases the flow of calcium* from brain cells, interfering with impulse transmission, changing brain function and causing confusion. The offspring of rats exposed for one month to 60-hertz electric fields simulating ground level under typical transmission lines, showed stunted growth, especially among males, as well as a higher mortality rate. ELF electric fields have also been shown to change brainstem levels of the neurotransmitter, acetylcholine.

Human cancer cells exposed to 60-hertz electromagnetic fields for no more than twenty-four hours experienced a six-fold increase in their growth rate one week later. Decreases in red blood cell counts as well as changes in the number and types of white blood cells have been observed in animals exposed to ELF fields. Thus, in summary, *ELF fields superimposed over man's natural bio-electric field can have serious negative biological consequences.*

Ionic calcium, the key regulator and producer of much of mans' bioelectric fields, is therefore seriously affected. Thus, some calcium-imbalance diseases may be *triggered by ELF fields from common household appliances.*

All of man's biochemical functions were developed under *the gentle influences of the solar system.* The earth's one gauss magnetic field has the effect of causing the pH of the extracellular fluids to "*gently rise*" similar to the effects of the magnetic beds, as bicarbonates and carbonates are converted to hydroxides and soluble carbon dioxide. For example, when water at a pH of 7.5 is passed through a 7000 gauss magnetic field, its pH dramatically increases to about 9.2 (See Table 10). Currently, one out of every ten Japanese and one out of every ten Germans are sleeping on magnetic beds and the phenomenon is beginning to spread dramatically throughout Europe. There are many thousands of well trained Western and Japanese doctors who sleep on these beds every night and swear to the benefits to health by doing so **Discovery of Magnetic Health,** by George Washnis,)

The Earth's magnetic fields, which affect our biochemical functions, have gone from *4 gauss* (magnetic lines per square centimeter) at the time of Christ to currently less than *1 gauss*. When, within a thousand years the Earth's magnetic field is 0 gauss, will we have to produce artificial magnetic fields to survive as a species. **(Note:** The Earth's magnetic field is generated by the electrical currents produced, electro-statically, by the mantle moving at a different speed than the molten core. When the mantle moves faster than the molten core, the flow of the electrical current, in a westerly direction, causes the magnetic pole to be in the north; when the mantle moves slower than the molten core, the flow of the electrical current, in an easterly direction, causes the magnetic pole to be in the south. When the mantle and core are moving at the same speed, no static electricity is produced and no magnetic poles exist. The torque on the Earth generated by its elliptical orbit through space and by the positioning of other celestial objects, dictates the changing speed of the mantle, and thereby the degree of the magnetic field and the *"flipping"* of the magnetic poles.) Also, the micro-pulsations of the moon, from 0.1 to 35 hertz (cycles per second) and the moon's orbital cycle of 28 days, are in perfect harmony with the electro-biochemical impulses that they helped to develop during the evolution of the human race; the most obvious being that a woman ovulates every 28 days. As well, of course, the sun provides the necessary radiant stimulus to the pituitary glands controlling the production of calcium regulating hormones, such as calcitonin, stimulating the body to produce, among other things, the calcium regulating inisotol triphosphate and the calcium absorbing vitamin-D.

Thus while the king of the bioelements, calcium, regulates the state of man's health, in order to be healthy, man must also be in harmony with the universe.

CHAPTER THIRTEEN

MEDICAL MISINFORMATION

Although these simplicities are obviously easy for you to understand, what you will find hard to understand is just how you are going to consume your seven full course servings of fruits and vegetables that are nutritionally required to maintain good health, every day. The only *realistic answer is dietary supplements*. Also, there are additional requirements which also must be met in order to remove the acidity of the body's fluids and maintain the required blue slightly alkaline pH of 7.4.

The first requirement, of course, is that the nutrients must be available for use by the body (see Table 4: Original Major Nutrients in the Body, and Table 5: Major Nutrients in the Blood). Our changing diets --- kids drink milk and adults drink beer, and our changing lifestyles --- kids play outside and adults work inside, can gradually erode our mineral nutrient stockpile to the point where *the body has to rob the Peter fluid to pay the Paul fluid*. There are many other, and more serious, changes which cause mineral deficiency to occur. Much of this has been caused by the misinformation propagated by the medical establishment.

One example that certainly must be contrary to God's intention is the familiar medical advice, *"Stay out of the sun,"* lest your skin produce the required vitamin-D to allow you to absorb the required mineral nutrients, thereby preventing disease. Another myth is, *"Adults do not need to drink milk,"* lest they keep their bones dense and ward off diseases like osteoporosis, arthritis, heart disease, and cancer. Besides, to get their required nutrients, the authorities could offer to let them do it the same way that the cows do it, and *"Let them eat grass."*   About 20 pounds per day would be required for human consumption. Other examples of the *don't eat myths* are as follows:

"Don't eat butter," so that you can avoid the natural nutrients of butter while allowing the substituted margarine to provide you with enough *cis-trans fats* to dramatically increase your harmful low density cholesterol levels (LDL's).

"Don't eat eggs," so that you can not only avoid consuming cholesterol, which has already been demonstrated in this book not to be the bad guy that it is made out to be, but by doing so, also avoid consuming **choline** which would make it difficult for your body to produce the neurotransmitter, *acetylcholine*, thereby helping to *induce senility*.

"Don't eat extra salt," as too much salt causes high blood pressure. However, a recent four year study by the prestigious Albert Einstein College of medicine (done in association with the prestigious Cornell University Medical college) on 1,900 men with high blood pressure, concluded that high blood pressure patients who ate less than 5 grams of salt a day had *more than four times as many heart attacks* as those who consumed over 10 grams a day. Although a *"tremendous"* increase in salt can lead to a *"small"* increase in blood pressure, low sodium causes the level of rennin hormone, secreted by the kidneys, in the blood to go up, and rennin is found in high levels of patients with high blood pressure. Thus, most Americans should double their salt intake.

"Don't eat vitamin and mineral supplements," lest you obtain all of the nutrients that your body requires for good health. Currently, 50% of Americans consume some minerals and vitamin supplements: 25% consume both of them on a daily basis. A 24 year study of 11,384 people by James E. Enstrom of the University of Southern California found that taking **vitamins and supplements cut the death rate in half.** Even more astonishing was the fact that deaths from cancers and heart disease for those taking the daily supplements was less than 10% of those who did not take the supplements. This study, by respected scientists at a prestigious institute of learning, of large numbers of people over a long time will be an excellent candidate for the AMA's waste basket, as rather than verify the results that are crucial to the health of America, the medical establishment will demand more proof as, while Americans are dying, it withholds funding for the studies.

There is other mis-information, which does not concern food, that is also propagated by the medical profession. For example: *"Your body temperature should not be allowed to rise above 98.6 degrees Fahrenheit."* What is left out is the phrase, **"for any length of time,"** as prolonged high body temperatures can, indeed, cause brain damage. But, what about short periods of time, and once again, why did **God in his wisdom** make humans suffer with fevers ? One answer is that many **viruses and bacteria cannot survive above the body's normal temperature**, and thus, the fever kills these critters. The doctor, on the other hand, is trained by the system to dispense an unnatural white chemical to quickly reduce the fever so that the virus can survive, thereby necessitating the other prescribed unnatural white chemicals, which are becoming increasingly ineffective, known as **antibiotics.**

Although the doctor's method of dispensing the drug industry's expensive chemicals has succeeded in the past, there is growing evidence that it will not always continue to do so, as many virus and bacteria have begun to develop an immunity or resistance to the antibiotics. But do not fret, as the drug industry is working on more, unnatural antibiotics as an answer to the problem, while medicine continues to ignore *God's intended, natural way*, such as garlic and onions in the daily diet. The natural antibiotics that they contain can kill both virus and bacteria, and were used extensively for surgery during World War One. The unnatural man-made antibiotics kill the weak virus first, making you feel good enough to stop taking the antibiotics. This allows the strong virus to live and grow stronger and eventually become resistant to the antibiotics. This does not happen with garlic and onions, as they are consumed daily, eventually killing the strong strain of virus.

Another mis-information myth is that *"Genes cause disease"*, the implication being that, because you are born with the genes that you have, there is nothing that you can do about the impending disease. But not to worry, because medical research is currently spending billions of dollars working on expensive ways to give you new, and healthy genes. The real tragedy with this situation is that it is *the acidosis that causes degenerative disease, and not the genes.* I'm sure that you're asking, *"If this is true, then what do the genes do ?"* The answer is that the *genes are the body's biological computer maps* showing the body which way it can go and can not go. Although they map the body's roadways to disease, they do not make the body go down any particular roadway. To put it in simpler terms, the genes dictate which of the many degenerative diseases to which you will be prone; they do not *cause* the disease. This concept, which is not understood by medicine today, is similar to the misconception that *the sun causes skin cancer*, when it is the *mineral deficiency induced acidosis* which *causes* the body to become prone to disease, and the genes only pick out which one of the diseases the body will be forced to choose. For some people, their genes are programmed to choose skin cancer.

The problem with propagating this last myth that " *God's sun is bad for you*," is that just the opposite is true. The sun shining on the body's skin does many positive things. One result is the photosynthetic production of the mineral regulator inositol triphosphate, *INSP-3*, an important biochemical mineral regulator. Another result of the sun shining on the skin is the photosynthesis of *vitamin-D* in the skin, resulting in increasing the small intestine's capability to absorb mineral nutrients, thereby *reducing the acidosis* known to cause degenerative disease. This includes *all cancers*. As researchers know, the acid in the fluids outside of, and inside of, the human cell can disintegrate the cell wall, allowing toxins and carcinogens to get inside of the cell. Dr. James P. Whitlock Jr., of Stanford University, describes carcinogens, such as dioxin, binding with receptor toxins inside of the cell to form molecules that are just the right shape and size to bind to the DNA's nucleotides. This causes the DNA template (structure) to bend or *mutate,* and *a cancer is born.*

Thus, the question of whether God's sunshine is good for your health is obviously so important that it should not be the responsibility of those making the claim that " *the sun is good for your health* " to prove the correctness of their claim to the governing medical authorities. The financial burden of further proof should be borne by the establishment. In fact, if the AMA is truly protecting the health of America, it should be responsible for financing the *third party* research to either prove or to disprove any medical claim. The assessment of the results should also be made by a *third party* group that does not have the same prejudice that burdens the current establishment, which is not only *judge and jury*, but also lavishes in the responsibility of being the *prosecutor*, or, in other words, "*three strikes and your out.*

For the sake of human health, *the burden of proof should be shifted to the well-funded establishment.* The onus should be on the establishment to prove, right or wrong, any claims made, for to fail to do so, will result in the suppression of legitimate medical advancements at a cost of great human suffering. One classical example would be the case of the association of disease to the acidity of the body's fluids. It has been scientifically established that, except for urine and stomach fluids, all of the healthy body's fluids are alkaline. If, as the top cancer researcher said, *"cancer cannot survive in an alkali"*, then cancer cannot survive in the healthy body's alkali fluids. Since the alkalinity of the body's fluids can be maintained by mineral and vitamin nutrients, this means that there is a means currently available to beat cancer, *inexpensive* nutrition, and that the search for an *expensive* man made chemical drug is the wrong way to go. As this book has shown, cancer is only one of many dreaded diseases that could be beaten by addressing the disease-nutrition issue. The stakes are too high to allow the AMA and the FDA to hide behind their feeble pass-the buck response of *"the burden of proof is on those making the claim"*. History has shown that scientific proof that does not conform to the establishment's preconceived concepts is *always rejected* initially; just ask Nobel Prize winners Max Planck, Albert Einstein, and Linus Pauling.

Also, the FDA has a terrible track record of prematurely approving drugs and then later being forced to take them off the market. For example, the following drugs were removed from the market in December 2000: *"Seldane"* (deadly interactions with other medications), *"Rotashield"* (bowel obstruction), *"Latronex"* (deadly intestinal effects), *"Resulin"* (deadly liver failure), *"Posicar"* (deadly interactions with 25 other drugs), *"Redux"* (heart valve damage), *"Hismanal"* (deadly interactions with other medications), *"Raxar"* (deadly irregular heartbeats), *"Trovan"*(liver failure), *"Duract"* (liver failure). These drugs approved and promoted by the FDA have now been proven to be *"deadly"* to humans. God save us from the FDA.

CHAPTER FOURTEEN

RECIPES FOR GOOD HEALTH

If the reader has made it this far, he or she has become somewhat familiar with the body's fluids, the human cell, the body's requirement for nutrients, and the body's *harmony with the earth*. The reader will by now understand that the <u>cause</u> of degenerative disease is *mineral deficiency* of the body, and the reader will therefore have a basic idea of how to both prevent and cure disease. But, unfortunately, knowing the basics is not enough, because most people want to be told, in simple terms, exactly what to do. Thus, what they want is science to give them a *recipe for good health*.

The first part of the recipe includes putting to use what you have learned in this book, so that your body has all the mineral nutrients it requires to maintain healthy, pH 7.4, body fluids. For example, the list would be as follows:

1.   Hipporates has been proven right, *sunshine is good for your health*. Don't be afraid of the sun. The sun should be one of your best friends. Although too much of anything is bad for your health, the same can be said for too little. Sunshine will

cause the photosynthesis of both vitamin-D and INSP-3 in your skin, both critical to human health, as they help raise the pH of the body's fluids, thereby helping to both prevent and cure disease. It will also induce *exitonic reactions* (see page 64) in your body fluids that will supply some of the energy required to maintain good health. Before the advent of artificial light, the human body, clothed in loincloth, was exposed to many hours of direct sunshine each day. This may have been too much. Less than one hour every day may be too little.

2. Not only is sunshine good for you, but also, *sunlight is good for your health*. Unfortunately, the artificial light has made a major change, for the worse, in human lifestyles. It is now possible to work and to live without sunlight using artificial lighting. The problem that this causes is that the body is moved from some of the *earth's nutrients*. Your hypothalamus and pituitary glands, located right behind the eyes, require unfiltered sunlight in order to regulate your appetite, sleep, body temperature, sexual functions, water balance, and hormones, many of which regulate body nutrients. All living things need to be *exposed* daily to sunlight. If a plant cannot grow healthy in its environment, then, in the same environment, neither will you. The human body should have at least one hour of unfiltered (preferably no windows or eyeglasses) sunlight every day, Hippocrates would definitely agree with this, as he stated that *"sunshine was good food and therefore good medicine "*.

3. Once again, Hippocrates' recommendation is correct, *fresh air is good for you*. This means you must get outside. Try taking a walk after every rain shower, or in the countryside if possible, while you are exposing yourself to your friend, the sun. As many pollutants, such as carbon monoxide, are heavy, the air is usually fresher at the top of a building than on the ground.

Table 11: Mineral Nutrient Content of some Popular Foods

Food (type)	Serving (amount)	calcium	magnesium	potassium
Yogurt, low fat	8 oz. cup	314	25	300
Orange juice, fortified	8 oz. glass	300	---	467
Milk, skim	8 oz. glass	302	33	382
Salmon, canned	3 oz. serving	167	25	272
Broccoli	4 oz. serving	108	---	478
Spinach	4 oz. serving	111	67	557
Banana	8 oz. (one)	11	95	770
Green barley essence	3 gm, teaspoon	33	68	264
Tomato	6 oz. (one)	5	19	491
Cheese	1 oz.. slice	174	15	198
Ice cream	4 oz. serving	100	12	150
Cabbage	4 oz. serving	51	19	273
Raisins	3 oz. serving	40	---	580
Pumpkin	8 oz. serving	60	---	500
Celery	2 oz. stick	21	6	158
Lettuce	2 oz. leaf	12	6	159
Green beans	2 oz. serving	25	---	110
Peas	4 oz. serving	29	12	150
Onion	2 oz. slice	23	5	78
Potato	8 oz. serving	30	---	334
Yams	8 oz. serving	20	---	340
Bread, 25% flour	1 oz. slice	20	8	40
Peanut butter	32 gm (2 tbsp)	10	---	210
Strawberries	4 oz. serving	20	---	60
Asparagus	2 oz. serving	10	---	110
Pineapple	6 oz. slice	15	---	138
Grapes	5 oz. serving	10	---	140
Prunes	1 oz. (one)	10	---	210
Rice	8 oz. serving	2	9	86
Corn	4 oz serving	4	---	314
Peach	6 oz. (one)	9	---	196
Apple	8 oz. (one)	7	---	105
Apricot	2 oz. (one)	5	---	100

Recommended Daily Consumption (RDCs)		2500	800	5000

Note: 1) Most nutritionists consider these listed foods as healthful.
2) Values will vary somewhat from producer to producer.
3) Foods at the top of the table have more minerals.
4) RDCs are author's personal opinion (for average adult)

4. Try to get outside close to the earth, as the *earth's magnetic field is good for your health.* Your body's natural bioelectrical system evolved under the influence of the overlapping magnetic field of the earth. Although the earth's magnetic field is very weak, so too are many of the body's bioelectric reactions; an example being the electrical requirement for the healing of wounds is only 0.00006 volts. Today, there are too many people who remain high in buildings most of every day, insulated from the earth's magnetic fields, Mother Nature's medicine.

5. Of course, once again Hippocrates has been proven right when he advised good food is good medicine: *eat lots of fruits and vegetables* (see Table #11: Mineral content of some popular foods). Both are full of vitamin and mineral nutrients, and both result in the production of alkaline salts that raise the pH of your body fluids, thereby helping to both prevent and cure disease. This may result in diarrhea some of the time, as some fruits and vegetables contain lots of the mineral nutrient, magnesium; however, remember, just as a fever is the body's way of killing virus and bacteria, diarrhea is the body's way of expelling toxins. Thus, *some fever and diarrhea can be very good for your health.*

6. *Don't eat more than 20 ounces of red meat each week, and avoid carbonated pop that contains high phosphates.* Most foods contain an abundance of phosphates, some dramatically more than others, and phosphates tend to precipitate out mineral nutrients causing them to pass out of the body, thereby resulting in mineral deficiency, which causes disease. Several major industries will be angry about this recommendation, but the facts are clear; diet can cause disease and diet can cause death.

7. *Eat white meat and fish.* White meat is both nutritious and low in the phosphates which cause mineral loss in the body. Fish is both nutritious and a rare source of edible vitamin-D.

8. *Eat nutritious natural foods such as butter and eggs.* Do not avoid these foods because of their cholesterol content, as to do so you would also be avoiding nutrients, such as choline, which are vital to human health. Besides, cholesterol is not the cause of heart disease, although, like all other foods, it should be consumed in moderation.

9. *Drink lots of milk, and dairy products*, as they contain lots of mineral nutrients and some are even fortified with vitamins. The most important critical nutrient is calcium, king of the bioelements. Everyone should drink milk, and when some do not, it is because their bodies are telling them not to drink the milk due to their state of acidosis. Although the bodies of such people are desperate for calcium, their bodies prefer to get calcium from a food that does not contain more of the acid, lactic acid, that is causing their acidosis. Thus they do not like milk. It's interesting to note that once the pH of the body fluids of these people is brought back to its normal alkaline level, they will start to crave milk. The body does know best.

10. *Drink the drink of princes and paupers, drink Kombucha* (see acids on page 120). Royalty drinks Kombucha because it works to prevent disease and maintain health. The poor commoner drinks Kombucha because it maintains health, it only costs a penny, and it tastes so good.   The nutritious organic nutrients are a powerful method of raising the alkalinity of the body's fluids, while dissolving toxins to which the Kombucha's gluceronic acid can then attach itself and expel from the body. This, in effect, is a great help to your liver and kidneys.

11. *Sleep on a magnetic bed or sit on a magnetic pad*, with the north, negative pole facing your body. This will cause the pH of your body fluids to become alkaline and cure your ailments.

12. *Get to know the nutrient content of foods that you eat*. Almost all foods currently list their nutrient contents on their packages. Table 11: Mineral Nutrient Content of Some Popular Foods should help get you started.

13. *Monitor your saliva pH and take vitamin and mineral supplements* according to Table 12: Recommended Daily Supplement Program. The saliva pH of children can respond positively to the program within days, the middle aged may take weeks to a few months, and the elderly may take up to a year or more to become a healthy caustic blue.

For those of you that *"just cannot take any more pills"*, the author recommends that you crush and pulverize them into a *powder* and include them in your natural foods. This can be done by putting a monthly supply of all of the dry vitamins and mineral supplements into a blender for about 10 minutes. This is a good idea as, although the calcium and magnesium tablets are in the readily ionizable carbonate form, it has been found that most of the one-a-day vitamin and mineral tablets can *pass through the bodies of the elderly in tact*. Thus, these tablets, *in double doses*, along with *a couple of trace metal tablets*, should be powdered with the calcium and magnesium tablets. Also, the vitamins A & D can be obtained in tablet form and added to the powder mixture resulting in about a *teaspoon per day* to consume. This teaspoon of supplements can be, for example, added to chocolate milk or cold fresh fruit juices, especially apple juice or Kombucha, for the

Table 12: Recommended Minimum Daily Supplement Program

pH	Calcium plus Magnesium		Vitamins-D + A	
6.5 to 7.4 (healthy range)	1200 mg (**3 tablets**)	690 mg	2400 IU (**6 tiny capsules**)	30000 IU
6.0 to 6.5 (developing a disease)	2400 mg (**6 tablets**)	1380 mg	4800 IU **(12 tiny capsules)**	60000 IU
4.5 to 6.0 (you have a disease)	3600 mg (**9 tablets**)	2070 mg	7200 IU **(18 tiny capsules)**	90000 IU

Note:

1) Calcium plus magnesium tablets, sometimes referred to as dolomite, weigh 1400 milligrams (mg) and can be purchased in large department stores, such as Walmart, for about 3 cents each. Each tablet contains 400 milligrams of calcium and 230 milligrams of magnesium. Each tablet may also contain trace zinc which is a bonus for your health.

2) Consumption of magnesium in amounts greater than 700 milligrams daily may cause stool to become soft (another bonus). If you are over this level, you will benefit from flushing the toxins out of your body.

3) The tiny (half the size of a pea) Vitamin A + D and round tablet or fish oil pills can also be purchased for just 2 cents each and contain 400 I.U. of vitamin-D, and 5000 I.U of vitamin-A.

elderly, or a milk shake for the kids. The presence of the *lactates* in the milk, or the *malates* in the apple juice, or the *organic acids* in the Kombucha, all allow the dissolved nutrients in the stomach to remain ionized, even when most of the stomach acids have been consumed and the pH rises. This allows the nutrients more time to be absorbed by the small intestine. The author also has found that the supplements taste good in both peanut butter and yogurt, but his personal favorite is to blend them with fresh fruit, such as cantaloupe, and ice in a high speed blender (*Vitamin-Fruit-Slush*).

(**NB:** The *Kombucha* mentioned above is a popular and nutritious drink, that only *costs pennies per glass*, that is consumed by *hundreds of millions of people each day*. It is made by the fermentation of a sugar tea mixture by a floating yeast fungi, known as the *"magic mushroom"*. All of the sugar is converted to a host of nutritious organic acids and the vitamins and minerals are liberated from the tea. The result after one week is a delicious, apple cider-tasting drink that has been consumed for hundreds of years by many cultures and has *more claims to health benefits than all of the claims for health benefits by other products combined*. The author believes the claims to be true, as he has found that the Kombucha helps to alkalize the body's fluids.)

Also worthy of note is a product that has been consumed by the Japanese for hundreds of years with a huge number of health benefit claims; it is known as *"coral calcium"*, and is currently being consumed by increasingly large numbers of people in the Western World. Coral calcium, the disintegration by-product of old coral reefs, is mined from old ocean beds at the base of the coral reefs of Okinawa. A significant amount of calcium, magnesium and other trace metals are dissolved by water. What this means is that the minerals are already ionized before entering your stomach. This is especially beneficial to *the elderly* who over time, *produce less acid*. This, combined with the bicarbonate anions in the coral calcium, Mother Nature's *milk of the ocean*, helps to keep the minerals *ionized longer* in the digestive tract. This leads to greater mineral absorption by the body.

One should remember that the consuming of calcium as a supplement is like consuming dairy products: the magnesium is like consuming vegetables (magnesium in the chlorophyll is what makes plants green), and the vitamin-A&D like fruits, vegetables and liquid sunshine. Also, *the vitamin-D dramatically improves the absorption of the nutrients by the small intestine.* Science has shown that, in the amounts recommended, these supplements cannot hurt you, but they can make all the difference to your health. Thus, Grandma was right when she said *"the secret of good health is milk, fruits, vegetables and sunshine"*. But, unfortunately, Grandma was only half right, as when God made the Earth and all its inhabitants, he used *all of the basic elements*, and most these basic elements are *sadly missing from our mineral depleted soils* and thereby our food chain. The first humans had all of these elements in their bodies. The water that they drank and the fruits and vegetables which they ate also contained all of these elements. The Biblical Patriarchs lived to an astounding old age: Adam lived for *930 years,* Methuselah for *969 years* and Noah for *950 years.* After the great flood covered their lands with nutrient depleted sand and clay, the Biblical Patriarchs did not live as long: Eber lived to *464,* while Issac only lived to *180* and Jacob to *147.* Today, except in rare areas of the Earth where degenerative disease does not exist and the average expectancy is 135 years, the soils, and, therefore, the foods grown in them, are depleted of most of these minerals and the life expectancy is half this. For example, the American doctor only lives for an average of *58 years,* while the average American lives almost two decades longer for an average of *76 years.*

The *common denominator* of the many cultures, who live to be 135 years old while maintaining a vigorous youth in *disease-free* societies, is that their soils are being *constantly replenished* with the mineral nutrients, most of which are missing in our soils. Except for some of the Japanese on Okinawa, all these societies all live in mountainous regions. They are the Tibetans, the Hunzas of Northern Pakistan, the Armenian, the Georgians, the Azerbaijans, the Vilcabamba Indians in Ecuador and the Titicacas in Peru, and a few other cultures. They all have their soils replenished with mineral nutrients contained in *the turbid water from melting glaciers*. The contained glacial-crushed minerals are so abundant that the water is white and is known as *"milk of the mountains"*. The islands of Okinawa were built up over the years from coral reefs. Rain erodes the coral reefs producing mineral rich *"milk of the oceans"*. All of these cultures also drink their water turbid. The contained dissolved minerals are so abundant that when they drink their customary four quarts each day, *"all"* of these disease-free societies violate our doctor recommended daily allowances, RDA's, by massive amounts. For example, they consume *70 times* the RDA of calcium, *22 times* the RDA of magnesium, *18 times* the RDA of potassium, *126 times* the RDA of iron, *120 times* the RDA of fluoride, and so on. And, to top it off, they continue to exceed these RDAs even further by eating foods which are rich in these minerals. Also they consume *"RDA unacceptable"* amounts of trace metals in their water while maintaining a killer diet rich in eggs, fat, milk, butter and salt.

The Hunza drink their 30 daily cups of tea, each with a large hunk of rock salt and two patties of butter. Our American disease- doctors, who die prematurely, ignorantly recommend that you *do not* follow the dietary example of the *youthful, energetic, and disease-free 135 year old Hunzas*. Nutrient trained veterinarians, on the other hand, have long recognized the importance of mineral, metal and vitamin supplements, and as a result, animal foods are full of these supplements. For example, horse food and dog food can contain as much as *60 nutrient supplements*. Meanwhile, human food remains almost totally depleted in these life sustaining nutrients. As long as the animals are fed only animal foods and not people food, they remain relatively disease-free.

Archeologists studying the cultures of the past 700,000 years have discovered that those who lived as hunting cultures had strong bones and were slim and relatively disease free, while those from agricultural cultures (starting 10,000 years ago) had weak bones, cavities and were disease prone. Diet was therefore the key factor. Agricultural cultures began consuming large amounts of carbohydrates which are readily converted to glucose. The pancreas must produce large quantities of insulin to convert the glucose into collagen and fat. The high insulin also causes the body to produce cholesterol necessary to construct new cells to store the fat. The result is high blood pressure, high cholesterol, acidosis from the sugar and fat storage. The hunting cultures are eating a high protein, low carbohydrate diet, resulting in a low glucose. This causes the pancreas to produce glucagon, which removes the fat from the cells to produce fuel for the body. The protein/carbohydrate (*procarb*) ratio of the disease free hunting cultures of the past was **1 to 1** (about 50% protein with 50% carbohydrates). In agricultural America today the procarb ratio is about **1 to 4** (about 15% protein with 60% carbohydrates). Noteworthy, the U.S.D.A recommends the **1 to 4** procarb ratio, which is the same diet used to *"fatten"* pigs. If the average overweight person would increase (for only 4 weeks) his protein and fat intake to 200 grams per day while lowering his carbohydrates to 40 grams per day (a procarb ratio of **5 to 1**), the pounds would drop off, muscle tone (shape) would improve, the insulin level would drop dramatically, the glucagon level would increase dramatically, blood pressure would drop, the cholesterol level would also drop dramatically, and toxins would be purged from the body. Every 4 weeks the carbohydrates can be increased by 40 grams until a noticeable gain in weight occurs. At this point reduce the carbohydrates by 40 grams per day and you will have determined your ideal procarb ratio (about **1 to 2**). Biologically, 10,000 generations are required to adjust to a major change in diet, but the human body has only had 500 generations to adjust from a natural procarb ratio of **1 to 1** to a procarb ratio **1 to 4**. The human body is therefore not currently designed for this **1 to 4** procarb diet, resulting in overworked organs (pancreas, liver and kidneys) and the inevitable diseases, such as diabetes and hypertension.

So, it appears that a procarb diet of **1 to 2** combined with high calcium intake is the answer. The question then becomes, is the consumption of liquid ionized calcium a good for you ? The answer is *"yes"*, *but only if you get about two hours of sunshine a day.* This will result in the parathyroid gland producing lots of the hormone calcitonin which will keep the serum (blood) calcium level normal, around the 100 ppm level, while inositol triphosphate, INSP-3 which serves to regulate the extraction of calcium stored in the cells, is photosynthetically produced by the skin. Those cultures that never get sick and consume 100,000 milligrams of calcium each day, practically live in the sun, and therefore produce adequate calcitonin and INSP-3, thereby maintaining a 100ppm calcium serum level in their blood, while regulating the proper amount of calcium to be stored in the cells. However, most of us do not get this amount of sun exposure, and as a result, the consumption of liquid ionized calcium can result in *"hypercalcemia"* where the serum calcium can reach as high as 200 ppm. In the book **"Warning! Calcium Deficiency"**, Kawamura and Taniuchi reported that a 30 year study with 20,000 case histories of over 40 over the counter calcium products, found that those taking liquid ionized calcium were suffering from acute hypercalcemia as evidenced by such symptoms as muscle weakness, polyuria, dehydration, thirst, anorexia, vomiting and constipation, followed by stupor, coma, and azotemia in severe cases. Due to the rapid increase of calcium in the blood, the kidneys will attempt to reduce the excess calcium by excreting it in the urine. This abrupt lowering of calcium may result in *"hypocalcemia"* causing muscle cramps, tetany, convulsions, respiratory distress, diplopia, abdominal cramps and serious metabolic disorders. However, the authors discovered that *over 30 years of study, none of the hyper/hypo-calcemic symptoms* *occurred with those in the 20,000 who ingested coral calcium or other marine calcium products.*

Richard Wood, Chief of the Mineral Bioavailability Laboratory at the Human Research Center at Tufts University in Boston, reports on 30 cases of calcium toxicity "from talking too much calcium over time". The symptoms were fatigue, dizziness, and soft tissue calcification. Of course, this is a very small group, and the hormone calcitonin, produced as a result of the sun striking the pituitary gland, could have prevented their hypercalcemia. Thus the problem was not excess calcium consumption, but rather, lack of exposure to sunshine. Also, according to this previously discussed massive Japanese study, had the thirty individuals been taking coral calcium, they would have never had problems with hypercalcemia, regardless of exposure to sunshine.

By now, despite the ignorant pleas from these doctors who go to their graves prematurely, you are probably wondering, "Where can I get some of this *Mountain Milk water,* or *Ocean Milk water ?"* The problem is that 100 % of the Mountain Milk water is consumed by these disease-free cultures. The more abundant Ocean Milk water is now available in America as *Coral Calcium.*
Unfortunately, having access to Mountain Milk water or Ocean Milk water for drinking purposes will not solve the problem of mineral depleted fruits and vegetables. The only answer would be to replenish our soils with all of the life sustaining minerals and trace metals so that we could begin consuming them in the produced food. Also, mineral and metal nutrients could be added to the water supply. Many believe that the addition of trace lithium, for example, to our water supply would dramatically reduce mental disorders.

However, this cannot happen overnight, and our health problems require immediate attention. Thus, until it happens, a man-made nutrient substitute with the right mixture of minerals, vitamins, and crucial trace metals (Table 13) will have to be provided. But this would be in violation of the laws in a society, such as America, which suppresses nutritional therapy and where *medical freedom,* (the *right to choose* and the *right to practice* the medicine of your choice) *does not exist.*

The amounts of supplements in the *recommended daily consumption* (RDCs), substantially exceed the ridiculously low RDAs set by the establishment, as does the actual consumption by cultures free of degenerative diseases, and, therefore, will be **_blindly_** condemned by our medical establishment. However, if God, or Hippocrates, the Father of Medicine, or your body were to be allowed to judge which is right, the RDCs found in the *Milk of the Mountains* and the *Milk of the Oceans* would be the clear-cut winner, *so claims the author !*

Table 13: Some Crucial Trace Metals

Metal	-----------------------Biochemical Purpose-------------------------
Boron	Needed in trace amounts for calcium uptake and healthy bones, and for the maintenance of normal levels of estrogen and testosterone in the blood.
Bismuth	Kills the bacterium **helicobacter pylori** which is proven to be the **"cause"** of peptic ulcers.
Chromium	Essential in the manufacture of cholesterol, fats and protein and maintains proper blood sugar levels and is therefore crucial in deterring diabetes.
Cesium	The largest and most alkaline metal, which, once inside the Human cell, cannot leave, thereby neutralizing the acids which " cause " the degenerative diseases, such as cancer, heart disease, arthritis, etc.

Table 13 Continued

Metal	----------------------Biochemical Purpose------------------------
Cobalt	Necessary for the production of the thyroid hormone, and is a crucial component of vitamin-B-12 which helps prevent anemia.
Copper	An important component of hundreds of human enzymes which help maintain the body's elasticity (youth), especially in the skin (preventing wrinkles) and in the cartilage and muscles and thus, helps to prevent aneurysms, arthritis, Cerebral Palsy, hernias, etc.. Also restores color to greying hair and is crucial for iodine utilization.
Germanium	Acts as a carrier for oxygen, similar to hemoglobin, and is therefore excellent at tissue oxygenation to help prevent viral infections.
Iodine	Crucial component of the thyroid hormone thyroxin which regulates heart rate, body temperature, digestion, general metabolism, body weight, the nervous system and reproductive system.
Lithium	Helps to dissolve kidney stones. Helps to control criminal behavior and depression. Lithium deficiency can lead to manic depression, reproductive failure, and reduced growth rate.
Manganese	Crucial component of many hormones, enzymes and proteins and is an activator for cartilage and bone development. Manganese deficiency can lead to deafness, asthma, Carpo Tunnel Syndrome and birth defects.
Molybdenum	Constituent of many crucial enzymes including aldehyde oxidase, sulfite oxidase, and xanthine oxidase
Praseodymium	Enhances the proliferation of normal cell growth, and in laboratory tests has **doubled the life** of some species of animals.

Table 13 Continued

Metal	----------------------Biochemical Purpose------------------------
Rubidium	The second largest and second most alkaline metal, which, once inside the human cell, cannot leave, thereby neutralizing the acids which **cause** the degenerative diseases such as cancer, heart disease, arthritis, etc.
Selenium	Selenium is the strongest metal antioxidant: it prevents cellular fats and lipids from going rancid and producing age spots and liver spots. It also helps to prevent heart palpitations, liver cirrhosis, sclerosis, cystic fibrosis, muscular dystrophy, multiple sclerosis, Alzheimer's, cancer, etc.
Silicon	Silicon helps keep fingernails and hair from becoming brittle while more than doubling the collagen in bone growth.
Tin	Helps prevent both hearing and hair loss while also helping to prevent cancer.
Vanadium	Enhances DNA synthesis and stimulates blood sugar oxidation helping to prevent diabetes.
Yttrium	Enhances the proliferation of normal cell growth, and in laboratory tests has **doubled the life** of some species of animals.
Zinc	Required for protein synthesis and collagen formation necessary for a healthy heart and healthy lungs, and promotes a healthy immune system and also promotes the healing of wounds.

CHAPTER FIFTEEN

CALCIUM AND ALLERGY

As was previously discussed, calcium ion influx is the trigger that causes the sperm and the egg to activate thereby creating life. Calcium in fact is involved in the regulating and governing of thousands of other biochemical reactions within the human body. In the case of allergy, it is a foreign substance or *allergen* that is the trigger for allergic reaction, with an influx of calcium ions into the cell quickly following. Now most readers would say, "Great, I'm getting calcium !" But the influx of calcium into specific cells is not always a good thing. For example, tumorous cancer cells are loaded with calcium, as is the plaque in plugged arteries. The question to be asked is "Where is the calcium coming from ?" In these two cases, as in allergic reactions, the calcium is coming from surrounding cells which were already calcium deficient, thus causing even further damage to these cells. What the body requires is a flood of calcium ions to fill the requirements of all of the body's cells. Thus, the influx of calcium into the cells, triggered by an allergen does not satisfy the body's need for calcium, but rather, just provides a chemical reactant, calcium (which is a crucial component of most biological reactions), that is necessary for the allergic reaction to proceed.

Although the exact *mechanism* of allergic reactions is well understood, the *cause* is not. More precisely, what causes the allergen to produce the allergic mechanism to occur in some people, while the same allergen is incapable of causing the same allergic mechanism to occur in other people ? The answer lies not in exploring the mechanism, or what happened, but rather in exploring why the mechanism occurred in the first place. To do so, an understanding of the biochemistry of the integral participant in the reaction, calcium, is required. But first, the allergic reaction mechanism itself should be explained.

There are three stages of an allergic reaction: **1.** sensitization, **2.** activation of the mast cells, and **3.** prolonged immune activity (*Allergy and the Immune System"*, Lawrence M. Lichtenstein, Scientific American, September, 1993).

The sensitization process is not thoroughly understood, but involves the reaction of interleukin-4 (secreted by the T-cell) with the remnants of an allergen that had been attacked by a macrophage. Wow ! These are big words. The T-cells are a part of the immune system that secrete chemicals to help defend the body against foreign invaders, such as viruses, germs and allergens. Interleukin-4 just happens to be one of these secretions. The macrophage is a large cell which latches on to and attacks these foreign substances. such as an allergen. The results of the interleukin-4 reacting with the remnants left over after being attacked by the macrophage is a B-lymphocyte plasma cell that is capable of secreting an allergen-specific molecule, *immune-globulin-E* or *IgE*. Thus, the *"antibody"* is born.

The second stage of allergic reaction involves the allergen produced antibody attaching itself to the cell surface of mast cells (a white corpuscle containing numerous, coarse, and irregular granules) in the tissue or blood. When an allergen comes into contact with two of the IgE molecules attached to the mast cell surface, it draws them together resulting in the activation of various enzymes (biochemical catalysts that stimulate chemical reaction) in the cell surface. The result is an influx of calcium ions, depleting the nearby cells of their crucial calcium stores, into the cell through the calcium channels in the cell surface, which then react with inisitol triphosphate, InP3, liberated from the inner cell surface. This induces chemically laden granules within the cell to become engulfed within the cell surface resulting in the discharge of chemicals to the fluids outside of the cell. The most well known of these chemicals is *histamine*. Drug companies have created several chemicals to counter the release of the histamine by the mast cell (anti-histamines) thereby alleviating the symptoms of the allergic reaction. Once the participation of the calcium in the allergic reaction is better understood, they will no doubt develop chemicals to "block" the influx of calcium into the cell thereby inhibiting the production of the IgE antibody. The result will be a body that is not cured, but rather, a body that is even more dependent on foreign chemicals and drugs.

The third stage, prolonged immune activity, occurs when the chemicals released from the mast cell induce the other cells in the blood to migrate into the blood vessel tissue (the walls of the arteries and veins) and contact external cells. The result is a host of activated cells that can leave the blood vessel tissue and expel tissue damaging chemicals.

Obviously, the "cure' for allergy can only come when we begin to understand "why" the IgE antibodies stimulate the influx of calcium into the mast cell. As was discussed in previous chapters, Dr. Reich had excellent success treating allergy patients as having calcium deficiency syndrome. Asthma, for example, was almost always virtually eliminated in children within days of treatment with vitamin-D and calcium supplements. Also, allergy symptoms were dramatically reduced in adults using the same treatment. Thus, another key factor is available to us in understanding the allergic reaction: that is that calcium deficiency plays a critical role in the allergic reaction.

The question thus becomes, how does adequate calcium in the extracellular and intracellular fluid affect the allergic reactions? It is interesting to note that in April, 2000, doctors at the university of Virginia discovered that the breath of asthmatics who are having an attack is 1000 times more acidic as normal. Although the exact biochemical mechanisms can only be speculated, there are many mechanisms that are already known as facts. For example, calcium deficiency causes body fluids to have a lower pH (or to become more acidic). Thus the allergic reaction must depend on a lower than normal pH. *Why ?*

One answer could lie in the fact that the rapid influx of calcium into the cell is pH-dependent: whether or not calcium flows into or out of a cell depends on electric charge differentials (between the inside cell fluids and the fluids outside of the cell) which are a direct function of pH differentials, as has been explained in previous chapters.

An abundance of calcium ions inside of the cell would raise the pH (or lower the acidity) thereby *reducing the electrical charge differentials* between the intracellular and extracellular fluids and result in the prevention of the flow of calcium in the calcium channels in the cell wall. Thus stimulation of the allergen by the IgE antibody would not result in a cascade of calcium ions into the cell. Thus, a major allergic reaction step would be dramatically reduced or eliminated. Also, the higher pH inside of the cell would cause the abundance of calcium already inside of the cell to be involved in other biochemical reactions, such as the production of nucleotides for DNA replication, and thereby be unavailable for participation in any allergic mechanisms. This also explains why, as mentioned in the Preface, Mr. Barefoot had noticed that his asthma attacks were inversely proportional to his exposure to sun, or in other words, they were dramatically reduced whenever he had a good tan. He also had noted as a young man that a tan prevented allergic induced hives.

When the vitamin-D receptors (VDR's) in the small intestine are saturated with vitamin-D, the body can increase its absorption of calcium 20 fold, thereby minimizing allergy. The sun is the best source of vitamin-D. In an article by P.C. Beadle entitled *"Cholecalciferol Production"*, Beadle describes how he measured the vitamin-D production in the epidermis (skin) to be 163 IU per square centimeter in light skin per day and 69 IU per square centimeter in dark skin per day. As the human body has 20 square feet of skin (18,580 square centimeters), the daily production of vitamin-D is between 1,000,000 and 3,000,000 IU, demonstrating that the recommended daily allowance (RDA) of 400 IU could be produced within 6 to 18 seconds of sunshine. This proves that the RDA for vitamin-D is ludicrously low. Evidence points to a prostrate, breast and colon cancer belt in the United States which lies in the northern latitudes. Rates for these cancers are two to three times higher than in the sunnier South. Thus allergy is also less prevalent in the South.

It therefore appears that allergy has the same cause as cancer and other major diseases. For example, it is well known that free radical damage of the brain is the main cause of Parkinson Disease. A free radical is a compound that has a shortage of electrons, and as a result is very positively charged. When the body has adequate vitamin-D (sunshine) and adequate calcium, the body fluids are alkaline and very negatively charged. Thus free radicals are destroyed upon entry into such a body, thereby preventing Parkinson Disease. It is interesting to also note that a study by the Albert Einstein College of Medicine reported in the April 2000 journal *Nature* that "free radicals have also been linked to the destruction of cells in diabetics triggering blindness, kidney failure and cardiovascular disease".

Thus, once again, natural nutrients, such as calcium rich foods and sunshine, can build up the body's natural defense mechanism helping to dramatically reduce both allergy and disease.

CHAPTER SIXTEEN

CAN CALCIUM CURE CANCER ?

In 1932 Otto Warburg won the Nobel Prize in Medicine for his discovery that cancer was anaerobic: cancer occurs in the absence of free oxygen. As innocuous as this discovery might seem, it is actually a startling and significant finding worthy of a Nobel Prize. What it basically means is that cancer is caused by a lack of free oxygen in the body and therefore, whatever causes this to occur is the cause of all cancers.

In chemistry, alkali solutions (pH over 7.0) tend to absorb oxygen, while acids (pH under 7.0) tend to expel oxygen. For example, a mild alkali can absorb over 100 times as much oxygen as a mild acid. Therefore, when the body becomes acidic by dropping below pH 7.0 (note: all body fluids, except for stomach and urine, are supposed to be mildly alkaline at pH 7.4), oxygen is driven out of the body thereby, according to Nobel Prize winner Otto Warburg, inducing cancer. Stomach fluids must remain acidic to digest food and urine must remain acidic to remove wastes from the body. Blood is the exception. Blood must always remain at an alkaline pH 7.4 so that it can retain its oxygen. When adequate mineral consumption is in the diet, the blood is supplied the crucial minerals required to maintain an alkaline pH of 7.4. However when insufficient mineral consumption is in the diet, the body is forced to rob Peter (other body fluids) to pay Paul (the blood). In doing so, it removes crucial minerals, such as calcium, from the saliva, spinal fluids, kidneys, liver, etc., in order to maintain the blood at pH 7.4. This causes the de-mineralized fluids and organs to become acidic and therefore anaerobic, thus inducing not only cancer, but a host of other degenerative diseases, such as heart disease, diabetes, arthritis, lupus, etc..

Everyone knows that the human body is made up of 78% water by weight, and that water is hydrogen and oxygen gases. When nitrogen gas and carbon in the form of carbon dioxide and methane gases are added, the total gas in the body by weight becomes over 95%. Almost half of the remaining 5% that makes up the human body and controls all biological functions is the mineral calcium.

No other mineral is capable of performing as many biological functions as is calcium. Calcium is involved in almost every biological function. This amazing mineral provides the electrical energy for the heart to beat and for all muscle movement. It is the calcium ion that is responsible for feeding every cell. It does this by latching on to seven nutrient molecules and one water molecule and pulls them through the nutrient channel. It then detaches its load and returns to repeat the process. Another important biological job for calcium is DNA replication, which is crucial for maintaining youth and a healthy body. Calcium ions are indispensable for DNA replication (*Calcium in the Action of Growth Factors*, W.H. Moolenaar, L.K. Defize, and S.W. Delaat, 1986 **Calcium and the Cell**, Wiley) which is the basis for all body repair. It can only occur *"on a substrate of calcium"* (*The Role of Calcium in Biological Systems*, Albert Lehniger, Professor of Medical Science, John Hopkins University, Volume I, CRC Press). Thus, low calcium means low body repair and premature aging. As important as all these and hundreds of other biological functions of calcium are to human health, none is more important than the job of pH control. Calcium to acid, is like water to a fire. Calcium quickly destroys oxygen robbing acid in the body fluids. Thus, the more calcium, the more oxygen, and therefore, the less cancer and other degenerative disease.

This information then begs the question, "How much calcium is necessary ?" Biologically, the human body requires 800 milligrams daily, but since calcium is extremely difficult for the body to absorb, the question then becomes "How much calcium do we have to consume to absorb 800 milligrams ?" As was discussed in previous chapters, the cultures around the world that consume "Milk of the Mountains", the Hunzas in Pakistan, the Armenians, Azerbaijans and Georgians in Russia, the Vilcabamba Indians in Equador, the Titicacas Indians in Peru, the Bamas in China and the Tibetans, all actually ingest an astounding 100,000 milligrams of calcium each day, and all have no cancer, diabetes, heart disease, arthritis, and all other degenerative diseases as well as mental disorders. This proves that you cannot consume too much calcium and that excess calcium must readily pass harmlessly out of the body through the urine. The only long living culture that does not consume the "milk of the Mountains' is the Okinawans who consume large quantities of "Milk of the Oceans"

Millions of Okinawans live in the southern coral islands of Japan with the average life expectancy of 105 years, while mainland Japan is just 77 years. The Okinawans live on islands made of coral reefs which are mainly calcium. The Okinawans discovered over 500 years ago that feeding coral sand that is produced from the weathering of the reefs to the chickens and cows results in twice as many eggs and twice as much milk. They also found that when the coral sand is used as a fertilizer, crops increase. by as much as three fold. When they finally, 500 years ago, began to consume the coral sand themselves, all of the under utilized doctors were forced to leave the islands. This was known in Japanese history as the Japanese Exodus.

The early European explorers discovered their secret and hauled shiploads of the calcium rich coral sands back to Europe. In Madrid Spain, the historic monument of the world's first drugstore contains rows of shelves labeled *"coral calcium from Okinawa Japan"*. Today millions of people all over the world consume coral calcium, and as a result, there are millions of medical testimonials.

The phenomenon of preventing and reversing degenerative disease through the consumption of large amounts of mineral and vitamins did not go unnoticed by men of medicine. Hundreds of years ago European doctors were prescribing coral calcium and other nutrients to their patients.

In the 1950s, Dr. Carl Reich M.D. discovered that his patients were able to "cure themselves" of almost all degenerative diseases by consuming several times the RDA of calcium, magnesium, vitamin-D and other nutrients. Dr. Reich was the first North American doctor to prescribe "mega doses" of minerals and vitamins to his patients and is considered by many to be the father of preventive medicine. By the 1980s Dr. Reich had cured thousands, but lost his license for explaining that the consumption of mineral nutrients, such as calcium, could prevent cancer and a host of other diseases. This concept was considered "too simple" to accept by the medical wisdom of the day. However, by the late 1990s, other medical men of wisdom were also discovering that calcium supplements could indeed reverse cancer. In the October

13, 1998 issue of the *New York Times* wrote an article appeared entitled *"Calcium Takes Its Place As a Superstar of Nutrients"* in which it reports that a study published in the *Journal of the American Medical Association* reported that "increasing calcium induced normal development of the epithelia cells and might also prevent cancer in such organs as the breast, prostate and pancreas". It also reported that the *American Journal of Clinical Nutrition* published "virtually no major organ system escapes calcium's influence" and that a research team from the University of Southern California found "adding calcium to the diet lowered the blood pressure in 110 black teenagers".

The January 14, 1999 issue of the *Phoenix Republic* wrote in an article entitled *"Calcium Reduces Tumors"* that the *New England Journal of Medicine* reported "adding calcium to the diet can keep you from getting tumors in your large intestine". Then the February, 1999 issue of the *Readers Digest* wrote in an article entitled *"The 'Superstar' Nutrient"* that the *Journal of the American Medical Association* published "when the participants consumption reached 1500 milligrams of calcium a day, cell growth in the colon improved toward normal (this means that the cancer was re- versed)". *The Digest* also reported that the Metabolic Bone Center at St. Lukes Hospital believes that "a chronic deficiency of calcium is largely responsible for premenstrual syndrome (PMS)" and that "a lot of women are avoiding the sun and their vitamin-D levels may be very low". In the same article, the Digest reported that "in 1997 the large federally financed trial found that a diet containing 1200 milligrams of calcium significantly lowered blood pressure in adults". Then the May 3, 1999 edition of *US World News Report* wrote in an article entitled *"Calcium's Powerful Mysterious Ways"*, that, "Researchers are increasingly finding that the humble mineral calcium plays a major role in warding off major illnesses from high blood pressure to colon cancer" and that "You name the disease, and calcium is beginning to have a place there" (David McCarron, a nephrologist at Oregon Health Sciences University).

Unfortunately, most doctors have not heard the news that their own journals, major newspapers and magazines are reporting that natural supplements, especially calcium, can cure and prevent disease.

The scientific evidence that calcium is the key to good and long health is overwhelming. Just 20 years ago, any doctor making the claim that calcium supplements could cure cancer would loose his license. Dr. Carl Reich lost his license for making this claim which the medical authorities of the day branded as *"too simplistic"*. Yet today, the doctor's own Journals: *The New England Journal of Medicine, The Journal of the American Medical Association*, and the *American Journal of Clinical Nutrition* are all making the claim that calcium supplements can reverse cancer and that virtually no organ escapes calcium's influence. These journals have been quoted in our popular and respectable newspapers and magazines. We have come a long way, and still have a long way to go. At present, it is almost impossible to find a doctor who is aware of these scientific findings. Therefore, we must get the doctors to read their own Journals and then do an almost impossible task, get the American Medical Association and the Food and Drug Administration to do their jobs and endorse these scientific findings. When this finally occurs, over 90% of disease will be irradicated thereby eliminating massive pain and suffering, and we will be well on our way to *curing America*.

One does not have to be a rocket scientist to read simple articles in reputable newspapers, magazines quoting the doctor's own journals that are all saying that disease can be cured by diet. Also one can simply look at the millions of people around the world that never get sick and say, "Lets do what they do!" Unfortunately, all of their milk of the mountains is consumed as fast as it is produced. However, the Japanese could cure the world with their "milk of the oceans" known as *coral calcium*, the calcium factor of good health.

CHAPTER SEVENTEEN

QUESTIONS AND ANSWERS

The most frequent question asked the author is, *"What do you do ?"* The response always begins with, *"I have not taken a pill in over 30 years."* Psychologically, taking pills is synonymous with taking drugs. Also, many people have difficulty swallowing pills. For most, many of the pills remain intact as they pass through the intestine undigested. The obvious solution is to do what the author does. First, the author puts all of the non liquid nutrient pills and capsules into a blender to make a pulverized blend. He then uses a flour sifter to remove the broken up oversized capsule containers. The author takes 24 pills and capsules each day, and he has found that when pulverized, the blend fills a heaping teaspoon. Thus the author pulverizes a three month portion and puts it into a large bottle labeled *"Hunza Powder"*, and then takes a heaping spoonful each day. Secondly, the nutrient blend should be taken at meal times, as for the elderly, this is the only time that they have sufficient acid in their stomachs to digest food. Thirdly, one glass of milk or one glass of apple juice should be taken with each meal so that the lactates or malates will keep the digested nutrients ionized even as they pass through the alkali duodenum, thereby allowing for greater absorption. Also, the consumption of fruits and vegetables with meals provides anions which enhance the absorption of nutrients.

The second most frequent question asked is, *"which are the 24 pills that you take ?"* The answer is 3 coral calcium (1.5 grams), 2 vitamin-D (5000 IU each), 6 multivitamins (one-a-day), 6 multi-minerals (containing 60 trace minerals), 3 calcium (citrate), 1 magnesium citrate, 2 vitamin-C (60 mg each), 1 vitamin-E (500mg), and 10 milligrams cesium chloride. The result is *Hunza Powder*. The author takes a heaping teaspoon each day, usually mixed in a fruit slush or a banana shake.

The next most asked question is, *"What do I have to do to cure .... ?"* The answer is that the body can cure itself of all disease if given the nutrients it needs. To begin with, the DNA which is the body's blueprint to cure itself and to stay young, only works *"on a substrate of calcium"*. Thus the DNA will only repair the body when the body fluids are full of calcium and therefore alkaline. This is why many diseases are considered to be incurable, as without nutrition, the body remains acidic and DNA replication is inhibited.

So then, what are the nutrients that the body need to cure itself. The answer begins with calcium. There is no such thing as a bad calcium nutrient. All calcium nutrients are good for producing a healthy body; however, some are better than others. For example, the consumption of coral calcium provides adequate calcium, magnesium and dozens of trace minerals for absorption by the body. Some calcium nutrients, such as calcium carbonate, are difficult for the body to absorb. This does not mean that they are not good, but rather that there are better choices. Also, there is no such thing as a bad coral calcium from Okinawa. They are all *miracle minerals*. However, some are better than others. The Japanese grade the coral based on magnesium content. The more magnesium a coral has, the higher it is graded. Consuming coral calcium can be classified in the same category as breathing as both fill the body with life sustaining oxygen. Most suppliers of coral calcium instruct you to take 2 to 3 capsules each day. But this is for *maintaining* good health. When you are sick, it is best to double-up to 4 to 6 per day. If you are really sick, with a disease such as cancer, Lupus, diabetes, etc., it is best to triple-up to 6 to 9 per day. The author has been told by many that a few months on the larger dose coral has successfully terminated their cancer, Lupus, Multiple Sclerosis and numerous other incurable diseases. Of course all of these people exposed themselves to sunshine and a host of other nutrients as well as the coral calcium.

Of course, other nutrients are also required, the most important being exposure to sunshine. Sun on the skin produces inisotol triphospate to regulate mineral disposition in the body and it also produces vitamin-D which allow the intestine to absorb large amounts of nutrients. The ultraviolet radiation from the sun striking the eyes stimulate the pituitary, pineal and hypothymus glands at the back of the eye to regulate the production of many hormones such as melatonin, seritonin and calcium-regulating calcitonin. Thus lack of sunshine on the body is responsible for a host of diseases, especially cancer. This sounds like a controversial statement, but not when you look at the facts. The cancer-free black African is naked in the sun all day while the black American, who avoids the sun like the plague, has three times the cancer rate of the sun worshipping white Americans. There is twice as much breast cancer in the Northern States as in the sunny Southern States. Prostate cancer goes up almost 300% from the sunny Mexican border to the Northern Canadian border. When exposure to the sun does trigger skin cancer, the victim is usually a white albino who already has five other mineral deficiency induced diseases, and is well on the way to developing the sixth.

Other important nutrient sources are multi-vitamins, which can be purchased inexpensively in all major stores. The instructions on the bottle may say to take one each day; however, the many cultures around the world that never get sick take about 100 times the amounts that is recommended in America. This means that you should take several every day, the author recommends at least 6 per day, as by the millions, these people have proven that there is no such thing as too much when it comes to vitamins and minerals. There is however, one exception, and that is large amounts of *liquid calcium* that can lead to hypercalcemia, if the body is not exposed to sunlight for at least one hour each day. Large quantities of coral calcium do not require sunshine as no amount of coral calcium can cause hypercalcemia. Also, trace minerals can be found in most health stores. Once again the instructions will say one per day, but 6 per day is recommended. Vitamin-D is also necessary to insure the absorption of nutrients. A minimum of 5000 IU is suggested. Extra boron, selenium, chromium, zinc, vitamin-A, vitamin-E and cesium is also recommended.

Although almost all degenerative diseases can be prevented and cured nutritionally if given enough time, people are always asking, *"What can I do if I am terminal ?"* A terminal cancer patient, for example, may be cured over a 6 month period by consuming the proper nutrients, but may only have 3 weeks to live. This situation requires a more potent nutrient treatment such as cesium chloride, for example. Cesium chloride is a natural salt, and where it is found, cancer does not exist. This is because cesium is the most caustic mineral that exists, and when it enters the body, it seeks out all of the acidic cancer hotspots, dousing the fire of cancer, thereby terminating the cancer within days. Also, when dimethyl sulfoxide (DMSO) is rubbed near a painful cancer, the pain is removed and the DMSO causes the cesium to penetrate the cancer tumor much faster, thereby terminating the cancer much faster. DMSO is an approved drug in 125 countries around the world and 600 million people have used it therapeutically. Larger doses of vitamin-D will cause the body to alkalize faster bringing a speedy end to the cancer. Otto Warburg's oxygen respiration enzyme formula (Oxy-Plus,   has also been proven to be effective against cancer. Dr Karl Folker discovered CoQ10 in the 1960s while working for the giant pharmaceutical company

Merck. He found it to eliminate cancer tumors in the breast, lung and stomach, *Biochemical and Biophysical Research Communications*, March 30, 1994. And finally, gold metal absorbed by the body has been found effective in recovering from cancer.

The following program has been found to be effective for cancer:

1. Consume 6 coral calcium capsules each day, 2 in morning, 2 in afternoon and 2 at night.
2. Consume 100 grams of cesium chloride at 3 grams each day (one gram morning, noon and night, total 33 days).
3. Consume 100 milligrams of CoQ10 each day for 30 days.
4. Consume one Oxy-Plus (500 mg) three times each day.
5. Apply DMSO gel to skin nearest the cancer (or nearest to pain) twice a day.
6. Apply gold gel to skin nearest the cancer once each day.
7. Consume 6 vitamin-D tablets (5000 IU) each day, 2 in the morning, 2 in the afternoon and 2 at night.
8. Eat two bananas, and/or two large potatoes, two glasses of milk or two glasses of orange juice and eat raisons, tomatoes, spinach or broccoli every day (all contain lots of potassium, magnesium and calcium).
9. Expose your skin and face to a least two hours of sunshine every day with no skin block and no glasses (allows for the production of inositol triphosphate, calcitonin and vitamin-D to help regulate crucial minerals such as calcium). Sun exposure is mandatory, even with skin cancer.

Note:

1. All of the above ingredients are available.
2. This program will help to alkalize the body's fluids, resulting in the toxins, which are adhered to the cell surface, detaching themselves and entering the blood. The body will recognize the toxins as foreign invaders and respond by attacking them possibly causing flu-like symptoms like headaches, stomach aches and diarrhea. This is called "detoxing" and it means that the body is ridding itself of cancer inducing compounds.

3. After the cesium has been consumed (33 days) the cancer will be benign (only a biopsy can prove this). Continue taking all of the other nutrients except for the DMSO which should only be used for pain control.

The author has witnessed numerous people with terminal cancers who have employed the above program successfully. In the author's web site (**www.cureamerica.net**), and in the Testimonials section of this book, numerous testimonials are provided by prestigious Americans. The author has also witnessed hundreds of other less prestigious Americans cure their incurable diseases. Although their testimony is considered hearsay and unscientific, examining their medical records, which state that they are all terminal, and then matching them to the now healthy bodies, is very exciting. Pancreatic cancer for example is a death sentence. When a tearful Ray explained that his mother was only given less that 3 months to live due to a metastasized pancreatic cancer, he readily defied his doctors and put her on the cesium program. That was 3 years ago and his mother recently remarried and is currently on her second honeymoon. A young lady in Oklahoma with metastasized cancer was scheduled for a double mastectomy and colonescopy prior to undertaking the cesium program. Today she is ecstatic as she has both breasts and her rectum is intact.

Alkalizing the body with nutrition allows the body to cure itself, even from previously incurable diseases. Nobel Prize winner, Otto Warburg complained in 1966 that because the agnostics were in control, millions of men and women would have to die needlessly from cancer. Today the agnostics are still in control, but their control has weakened substantially, due to information exchange by computers and the internet. The time is ripe to end the needless suffering, pain and death caused by curable degeneration diseases such as cancer and heart disease. The time has come to *"cure America"*.

CHAPTER EIGHTEEN

Coral Calcium and Microbes

*In the beginning of time when life
began in the ocean, one of the most
primitive organisms was coral.*

*Coral reefs are formed over thousands
of years with thousands of different corals.
Some reefs build up into islands like Okinawa.*

*These reefs are gradually worn away by the waves and
the weather. The ground up coral sinks to the seabed
where it mingles with the water and its contained
mineral and plant life.*

*Over millions of years the coral is bio-chemically
altered to contain all of the mineral nutrients of the sea
as well as its original nutrients of life. The result is a
power- house of natural marine nutrients known
around the world as,*

"coral calcium"

About 80% (four fifths) of the total animal life on the planet exists in the seas. Plant life is also abundant and seaweeds, especially kelp, are among the fastest growing most prolific plants on earth. The biomasses vary in density throughout the ocean. The deepest parts of the ocean supports life forms about which we know very little. Whilst we are still exploring the landmass of the earth, the oceans hold many secrets that are relatively inaccessible. This under-explored frontier of waters of the worlds surface has a volume of 42 million billion cubic ft or 286 million cubic miles, containing all of the elements found on Earth, and in amazing amounts.

Experts believe, for instance, that the average gold content is 0.012 parts per billion. This calculates out to be 460,000,000,000 ounces of gold or over 100 times the gold currently held in all the world's vaults. When gold is present in the soil, which is usually the case, it accumulates in the plant's protein and chlorophyll. The roots of plants can even break up rock, liberating the gold for uptake by the plants. When animals eat the plants, gold accumulates in the proteinaceous substances, such as hair, liver, brains and muscle. Man not only eats the bread made from the golden wheat, he also eats the animals who ate the gold. In many countries, gold leaf is popular in the diet. Gold is found in man's liver, brain and muscle and human blood has been measured at 0.8 parts per billion, and 43 parts per billion have been found in human hair. Human feces and urine have been known to contain startling amounts of gold: the ash of human excretion has been known to contain 1/3rd of an ounce per ton or over 10,000 parts per billion. The fact that gold exists in the human body in such significant amounts means that is must serve a useful function. Gold has been used successfully in some cancer treatments. Gold suspended in gel has also been used to treat wounds, resulting in rapid recovery and minimized scaring. There are hundreds of industrial processes where gold is used as a catalyst, and one day man is certain to discover that gold serves as a crucial biological catalyst in the human body. Thus, the oceans are an enormous collection of metals, minerals and chemical substances that sustain life. The seas contain many factors that are produced by its own living organisms.

The chemical balance in the oceans supports life in complex ways. Therefore, one cannot be surprised by scientific reports that many marine life forms and their environmental waters or habitants, such as coral reefs, produce substances that have potent and versatile biological actions in nature. Marine compounds of various types have been found to be antifungal, antibiotic, anticancer, antiviral, growth inhibiting, and analgesic.

Coral reefs are sea mountains of minerals of which calcium carbonate predominates, along with numerous other inorganic and organic forms of calcium. Calcium is a biological glue and an inorganic building block that is ubiquitous on the planet earth. In order to build a reef, the living coral polyps require specific climatic and ecologic conditions. Indeed, coral reefs are most preponderant in warm shallow waters of the ocean which have a range of temperature from 20 ° C to 30°C, approximately. Without sunlight the living infrastructure of organisms on the reef that use photosynthesis for nutrition cannot survive. These photosynthetic organisms, algae, are quite primitive, but efficient in forming a basic nutrient source for the food chain of the reef dwellers. Some marine organisms rely heavily on the photo-synthesizing organisms. The most interesting aspect of coral is their efficient and versatile ability to reproduce. They can reproduce by budding in an asexual manner and many polyps can form with remaining connections to its forerunner. Once a year, the corals may spawn filling areas of the reef with *massive amounts of eggs and sperm* (the reefs are submerged in a cloud of sperm and eggs) which attract plankton eating fish and mammals.

The basic photosynthetic organisms and plant life provide food for vegetarian inhabitants such as damsel fish, parrot fish, blennies and puffer fish. The parrot fish play a unique role in the biomass of reefs. They use their strong teeth to chew away as coral which is ground in their digestive tract and released to form the grand-up, sandy bases of the reef. In fact, parrot fish and similar *"coral munchers"* are a prime source of marine coral that is harvested as coral calcium.

It is clear that the geological evolution of Okinawa and its adjacent islands affects the environmental availability of minerals. The islands are composed of about 60 land masses of variable size that form an arc in the ocean, spanning several hundred miles. The largest land masses are volcanic in origin with raised profiles, but the coral islands tend to be flat. A unique feature of this geography, that may account for even more abundance of various minerals, is the *"proximity of coral reefs to volcanic material"*. Volcanic material forms soils that are exceedingly rich in trace elements, resulting in and even greater source of minerals that are incorporated into Okinawan coral (see Tables 14 and 15). Thus the coral from Okinawa is dramatically chemically different from all other corals. In addition, its marine microbes are specific to the islands of Okinawa, and are not found in other corals. Thus Okinawan coral is uniquely different from all other corals.

Table 14 lists the parts per million of the main elements found in fossilized corals. A detailed break down of the mineral profile of coral is shown in Tables 14 and 15. It is apparent that almost every natural element known to man finds its way into stony coral over the many years of growth of the reefs. The chemical analysis is always expressed as whole rock analyses which, if accurate should add up to about 99% with the 1% balance being composed of trace elements (see Table 15).   The elements are expressed as oxides with the loss on ignition (the weight loss when heated to 1000 degrees Centigrade) representing the gasses lost upon heating; water, carbon, nitrogen and sulfur.

<u>Table 14</u>: Major Elements Found in <u>Marine</u> Coral Calcium
– certified "whole rock" analyses, R. Barefoot.

Assay	Per Cent	PPM Metal
Silicon Dioxide	3.92	18,318
Aluminum Oxide	0.32	1,693
Calcium Oxide	33.60	240,000
Magnesium Oxide	18.90	114,000
Sodium Oxide	0.42	3,360
Strontium Oxide	0.33	2770
Iron Oxide	0.14	979
Loss on Ignition	41.3	
Total Majors	**98.93%**	

<u>NB:</u> Loss on ignition is the total of water , carbon, nitrogen, sulfur

Table 15:   Trace Elements Found in Coral Calcium
-certified "trace" analyses" by R. Barefoot
*-adapted from Bhalstead, MD1999

Elements	Result (ppm)	Elements	Result (ppm)
Aluminum	1693	Manganese	20
Silver	7	Molybdenum	<1
Arsenic	trace	Niobium	<1
Barium	10	Nickel	7
Boron	1	Phosphorus	280
Bismuth	4	Potassium	830

Cadmium	trace	Lead	trace
Cobalt	11	Rubidium	20
Chromium	80	Antimony	<2
Cesium	20	Selenium	14
Copper	23	Strontium	2770
Iron	979	Yttrium	3
Iodine	9	Vanadium	20
Hafnium	<1	Tungsten	0.1
Mercury	0.01	Zinc	16
Lanthanum	2	Zirconium	<1
*Bromine	0.14	*Osmium	<0.2
*Deuterium	150	*Palladium	0.025
*Dysprosium	0.18	*Platinum	<0.03
*Erbium	5.19	*Praseodymium	2.73
*Europium	<0.1	*Rhenium	<0.2
*Gadolinium	0.094	*Rhodium	<0.02
*Gallium	0.692	*Ruthenium	0.081
*Germanium	0.191	*Samarium	<0.05
*Gold	<0.05	*Scandium	0.049
*Holmium	0.091	*Sulfur	1780
*Indium	<0.06	*Tantalum	<0.01
*Iridium	<0.04	*Tellurium	<0.02
*Lithium	0.66	*Tin	0.198
***Lutetium**	**0.78**		

Next to calcium, iron is the most abundant mineral in the human body, crucial for maintaining oxygen. Coral calcium is a rich source of iron, containing almost 1000 ppm. Iron permits effective oxygen transport and storage in muscles and the blood. It is the central component of hemoglobin in the red blood cells. Iron deficiency causes anemia and abnormal fat metabolism. Iron competes with other elements for absorption into the body (competition with magnesium, copper, calcium and zinc).

C enhances iron absorption and classic consequences of iron deficiency are weakness, fatigue, poor immune function and anemia. The common belief is that *"too much iron can be toxic"*. The problem with this is that the words *"too much"* have never been defined. Also, United nations Health agency, UNESCO says that the majority of American women are anemic, as a result of iron deficiency. Although the RDA for iron is 18 mg/day of iron, many nutritionists advocate at least 40 mg/day. The full term infant requires 160 mg, and the premature 240 mg during the first year of life. The 240 mg at the average 5% absorption when consumed equals 4800mg/year or 13 mg/day for the first year of life. The RDA for an adult is 18 mg/day. Also, for pregnant women, there is a requirement of 1mg/day in menstruating females. At 5mg/day this is 20mg/day consumption. Pregnancy also increases demand for iron. Expansion of the mother's red blood cell mass requires 400 mg of iron, and the fetus and placenta require an additional 400 mg iron. Blood loss at delivery, including blood loss in the placenta, accounts for another 300 mg iron. The total requirement for a pregnancy, therefore requires about 1100 mg iron. At 5% iron absorption, this works out to 90 mg/day consumption requirement for a pregnant woman, but the RDA for an adult is only 18 mg/day. Thus, most women in America are being poisoned by iron deficiency.

The human body is only capable of absorbing about *800 milligrams of calcium each day*. Unfortunately, calcium is one of the hardest minerals for the body to absorb. Many of the calcium supplements are only in the 2 to 3% absorption range, while the so called *"great"* supplements are about only 15%. The cultures like the Hunzas, who consume over 100,000 mg of calcium each day obviously get their 800 mg absorption, while harmlessly passing the rest in their urine and excretion. With the Okinawans, because of the microbes in the coral, discovered by Swedish scientists in the 1990's, the absorption approaches nearly 100%. Therefore, taking a 250 mg of calcium in an antacid product, which does severe harm to the elderly by wiping out there crucial stomach acid supplies, usually results in the absorption of 5 mg (2%) calcium by the body over a 20 hour period. Also, there is substantial evidence that the nutrients in coral are *absorbed in less than 20 minutes* (the blood chemistry undergoes a drastic change, for the better, in less than 20 minutes). Therefore the 250 mg of calcium in the coral results in 250 mg being absorbed by the body in less than 20 minutes, and without destroying the crucial stomach fluids. That's almost *"50 times as much calcium, 50 times as fast"*. No wonder the coral calcium works so well ! In addition, when people have major diseases, the consumption of a triple dose of coral provides the maximum calcium absorption.

Coral calcium was first introduced to Western culture when it was brought to Europe by the Spanish explorers about 500 years ago. The world's oldest drugstores in Spain, which today are historic monuments, have clay pots on their selves labeled *"Coral Calcium, Okinawa Japan"*. Literature written by doctors of the day told of miraculous cures. By the turn of the 20th Century, the consumption of coral had spread to mainland Japan, where currently there are about 17,000,000 users. Today there are millions of consumers in China, Russia, Britain, France and Sweden. When coral calcium was brought to the Western communities as a *"modern"* dietary supplement in the 1970's, much misunderstanding was propagated by marketing companies. There is a *naïve notion* that when coral calcium is added to water it should dissolve completely. I am often asked about this circumstance, but the answer is obvious. If coral were soluble in water completely there would be no coral reefs in the oceans!

The reason why this question is asked often relates to the popular use of coral sand in tea bags which are merely added to water and the water is then consumed. Whilst coral calcium tea bags can import desirable properties to water, such as the transfer of important marine microbes, taking coral calcium in this manner is far less desirable then consuming the whole coral in powder or capsule form. Tea bag coral is less effective, as the user is only benefiting from about 2% of the marine nutrients that dissolve and the consumer, unless told, is almost unaware that he is consuming coral water, than a valuable way of obtaining the full benefits of coral calcium when it is consumed in its complete format, resulting in the consumption of over 50 times as much mineral nutrients. Also, the marine coral that is totally consumed is rich in the required nutrient, magnesium, as well as richer in all other nutrients.

Fossilized coral that has been washed up onto beaches has lost some of its mineral content by weathering and it may be dried and finely powdered to make a quick change of water pH. In addition, some commercially available coral calcium products have calcium added in hydroxide forms to increase alkalinity. Also, fossilized coral contains less than 1% magnesium, whereas marine coral has about 12% magnesium, which balances the 24% calcium for a perfect biological 2:1 calcium/magnesium ratio. Because of this lack of magnesium in fossilized coral, magnesium compounds are often added, resulting in a substantial dilution of the coral. After studying many types of coral supplements, I have concluded that marine coral, not fossilized coral, taken in complete format is obviously the most ideal way to consume coral calcium for health.

As a result of competition, those selling fossilized coral mislead the public into thinking that because they remove their coral from the beaches they are not harming the coral reefs, implying that those *"mining"* the marine coral must be harming the reefs. The truth is that the *"harvesting"* of the marine coral is done under the strict supervision off the Japanese Government who enforce, by jail incarceration, if the slightest damage occurs. In reality, the deposition of the coral sands (coral calcium) at the base of the reef actually inhibit the growth of the coral reefs. The islands of Okinawa are very shallow with little wave action allowing the coral sands to pile up, choking off the reef. In places like Hawaii, where there is lots of wave action, the coral sands get washed out into the ocean. When the coral sands are removed by harvesting, the reefs come alive and flourish. Thus harvesting marine coral calcium is not only beneficial to man but to the coral reefs as well.

Many commercial companies have promoted coral calcium from Okinawa as though it is all the same material. However, the harvesting of marine bed coral calcium is much more difficult and costly than merely collecting fossilized coral from beach mines. This fossilized coral has undergone thousands, if not millions, of years of erosion, loosing most of its magnesium content and much of its trace metal nutrient content. Also, because of the hype generated by coral calcium testimonials, numerous, unscrupulous entrepreneurs are harvesting coral from other locations around the world (this coral does not have the desired microbes), but telling their customers that it comes from Okinawa. Some even go so far as to blend their coral with Okinawan coral so that they can make the claim that it comes from Okinawa.

In my studies of the selection of different types of coral, I have learned that careful selection of a suitable grade material is necessary. Therefore, I was horrified to find some commercial types of coral calcium that were less than 10% coral calcium. This practice has emerged in the manufacture of some types of coral calcium capsules. The addition of inert magnesium or calcium should be disclosed by manufacturers on their labels. The public should look for a label that declares a minimum of *"1000 milligrams of coral calcium"*, content (from Okinawa) *in a daily dose* preferably *"marine coral"*. Many of the diluted versions have less than 500 milligrams of coral calcium per daily dose. As mentioned earlier, marine based or fossilized coral calcium does

156

not provide alone enough magnesium to meet recommended magnesium levels for health. This is why, I have stressed nutrition with high magnesium and mineral diets as an important factor in health maintenance. After all, we use the term dietary supplement and it must be understood that supplements are not to be confused as alternatives to a healthy balanced diet. The word *"supplement"* implies extra nutrient ingredients to provide health benefits over and above a balanced diet.

D espite the deficiencies, both tea bag coral and fossilized coral consumption has led to remarkable health testimonials, although not as many as the consumption of marine coral. This is due to the *"microbe factor"* (explained in detail in the next paragraph). In addition there are many other factors that make coral calcium of marine origin more ideal for health. I prefer coral that is used in vegetable capsules or at least capsules that are made to dissolve at the right time to provide the best circumstances for mineral absorption. The practice of breaking capsules and adding the contents to water is unnecessary, except in circumstances where some people cannot readily swallow capsules.

M icrobes or bacillus are defined as any genus of rod-shaped bacteria that occur in chains, produce spores and are active only in the presence of oxygen and water. Although some microorganisms are destroyed in the process of drying, this process is not *per se* lethal to microorganisms. The addition of water can spring them back to life. Microbes can be found living in all living animals and plants. Of course most microbes can live off of plants and food, and are best known for their ability to *"spoil"* the food. Actually *spoiling food is a form of digestion*. Thus spoiled food is pre-digested by the microbes. This is probably the reason that most of the animal kingdom, including humans, have substantial numbers of microbes in their intestines. The strong acid in the stomach can not break down all food, especially complex carbohydrates. However, the microbes in the intestine living off of these foods, do indeed break them down and make them available for absorption by the small intestine. Also, the rod-like shape, allows the microbes to penetrate deep into the *"finger-like villi"*, 5,000,000 lining the intestine, where they can easily be absorbed by *1) facilitated diffusion* (glucose combines with a carrier substance which is soluble in the lipid layer of the cell membrane), *2) osmosis* (the movement of water molecules and dissolved solids through semi-permeable cell membranes from an area of high concentration to an area of low concentration), *3) filtration* (movement of solvents and dissolved substances across semi-permeable cell membranes by mechanical pressure, usually high pressure to low pressure), *4) dialysis* (separation of small molecules from large molecules by semi-permeable membrane) and *5) pinocytosis* (or "cell drinking" where the liquid nutrient attracted to the surface of the cell membrane is engulfed). As a result, the *"microbes are crucial to life"*. Fortunately, most of the hundreds of non-marine microbes found in the human intestine were transferred by the mother. Some animals, like the baby elephant, have to eat their mother's excrement just to get the needed microbes.

The genera of bacteria that are found in the intestinal tract are: Bacteroides (22 species, non-sporing rods), Clostidium (61 species, heat resistant spore-forming rods), Citrobacter (2 species, lactose fermenting rods), Enterobacter (2 rods, ferment glucose and lactose), Escherichia (one specie, rods), Lactobacillus (27 species, non-sporing rods employed in the production of fermented milks), Proteus (5 species, aerobic rods that hydrolyze urea), Pseudomonas, 29 species, most important bacteria in spoilage of meats, pultry, eggs and seafoods), Salmonella (1800 species that ferment sugars and glucose), Shigella (4 species, aerobic, like pollutuon), Staphylococcus (3 species, coagulate blood, also common in nasal cavities) and Streptococcus (21 species).

Salt greater than 1% can cross the cell membranes of most bacterium by osmosis, which results in growth inhibition and possibly death of the microbes. Everyone is also familiar with the preservation of meat by *"salting"*, which kills or inhibits the bacteria. Thus large quantities of salt in the intestinal tract, which occur when large quantities of nutrients have been digested (hydrochloric acid from the stomach reacting with the sodium bicarbonate from the pancreas produces salt in the duodenum), can kill the microbes, thereby inhibiting nutrient absorption by the body, especially when large amounts of nutrients have been ingested..

On the contrary, *"marine microbes"*, such as those found in coral calcium by the Swedish, thrive in high salt environments Also because of their original salty marine environment, as well as their calcium magnesium and mineral environment, the marine microbes have no difficulty assisting the body to absorb high quantities of these minerals, especially when the intestine is saline, resulting from the consumption of large amounts of mineral nutrients. These same salts, however, incapacitate the natural microbes in the intestinal tract, thereby inhibiting nutrient absorption. Thus, the coral marine microbes resolve this problem, dramatically increasing the absorption of the nutrients by the body.

Those people using a small sachet teabag that allows only a tiny amount of coral to dissolve in the liquid in which they are placed, and those using fossilized coral, still get some benefits from the marine microbes, hence the testimonials. Also, these testimonies emanating from the small intake of nutrients is nothing short of astounding. The reason, for this success is that when the teabag or the fossilized coral is placed in a liquid the microbes come to life and are consumed when the liquid is drank. These microbes can then latch on to nutrients already in the duodenum and pull them into the body resulting in health benefits. Consumption of marine coral, on the other hand, allows the *"total nutrient content of the coral"* to be consumed as well, and therefore provides far greater health benefits, leading to more testimonials. The bottom line is that all coral from Okinawa has fantastic health benefits, but the ***marine coral is far superior***.

Coral is also very much like human bone and the body does not reject it, and it is conducive to allowing new bone growth. In Germany, surgeons will pack the cracks and holes in the broken bones of the elderly with a coral paste made from coral calcium and water. Within 3 weeks the coral is displaced with new bone growth. James Tobin in the Detroit News writes that *"because of a gift from the sea, coral calcium, Christian Groth is swimming again'.* The coral rests snuggly inside the femur (thigh bone) of his right leg, just above the knee. It fills a hole the size of a large marble, replacing a benign tumor that was making it harder and harder for Chris, 14, to play the sports he loves. If you use a powerful microscope to compare the coral to Chris' bone, you could not tell the difference. Chris is one of the first people in Metro Detroit to have a bone repaired with sea coral and is *doing everything"*, said his doctor, Ronald Irwin, an orthopedic oncologist affiliated with the Beaumint Hospital, Royal Oak. *It looks good,"* Irwin said, *"he'll ski this year !"*

In the May issue of the New England Journal of Medicine, 2001, wrote about the ***"bionic thumb"***. Doctor Charles Vacanti at the University of Massachusetts re-created a thumb for Paul Murcia who had lost his thumb in a machine accident. First a small sample on bone from the patient's arm bone was cultured to multiply. Then a sea coral scaffold was sculpted into the shape of the missing thumb bone, and then implanted into Murcia's thumb. The patients own bone cells, grown in the lab, were then injected onto the scaffold. The bone cells grew a blood supply and the coral scaffold slowly melted away leaving a new living thumb bone. The doctors predict that eventually all that will be left will be a thumb bone with healthy bone cells and no coral. 28 months after the surgery the patient is able to use his thumb relatively normally and the doctors say that the experiment in tissue engineering using the coral is working.

One must be naturally suspicious of any dietary supplement or factor that appears to have such panacea benefit. In the case of *"coral calcium"*, this versatile benefit that has resulted in literally millions of testimonials over the past 600 years is explained by the varied quantity of minerals contained within the coral (as a result of the coral leaching nutrients from the ocean waters for millions of years) and their important role in the maintenance of almost all important body structures and function, as well as the beneficial results of injecting the contained marine microbes into the human digestive system.

Scientifically, all testimonials are considered as hearsay and are inadmissible. The same is true in our courts. However, when the number of testimonials becomes significant, so to does the content of the testimonies. Coral calcium has a track record of well over 600 years, with testimonies about health benefits from the very beginning. It was these testimonies that induced the Spanish explorers 480 years ago to fill up their ship holds with the coral calcium and to return to Europe where the testimonies continued, and have done so to this very day. Japan, China, Russia, Sweden, France and England have tens of millions of people taking coral calcium daily with reportedly millions of testimonials. Coral has only been in America for a few years, but already the testimonies are flooding in. Here are a few examples:

TESTIMONIES:

#1.   Hello, my name is Conrad Sims, I am 29 years old and I live in Decatur, Ohio. I am athletic and consider myself to be in good health. A few months ago my neck began to get sore and then began to swell. I tried to ignore it, but it began to become painful. It was not long before the swelling was the size of a golf ball and my co-workers demanded that I see a doctor. It was diagnosed as ***malignant cancer*** and the doctor told me that it had to be removed surgically. He said there was no other way. I did not have health insurance for the surgery and I was terrified. A friend suggested I try coral calcium. I thought "what's a little calcium going to do for me ?" I was desperate so I started taking the coral and within a week the pain had subsided. After two weeks the size of the tumor was dramatically reduced, and after four weeks it appeared to be gone. I am back to my old self and feeling great.

God bless coral calcium, Conrad Sim. (March, 2001)

#2.   My name is Sue Ann Miller and I live in Akron, Ohio. I had been suffering for years with several diseases: ***diabetes, Bells Palsy, carpel tunnel syndrome***, and I have had hip knee and elbow replacements. I lived on drugs and was in constant pain. I could barely walk and could not climb stairs. Then my sister went to a talk by Mr. Barefoot and brought me some coral calcium. I was in such pain and was so desperate that I would try anything. In just a few weeks the pain went away. A few weeks later and I returned to full mobility as my swelling went down and my hands straightened out. A few weeks more and I could bend over, touch my toes and run up stairs. I have gotten my life back. The coral was magic and I thank God for the coral and Bob Barefoot.

I love you all, Sue Ann Miller, Ohio

#3. My name is Donna Crow and I am struggling to recover from *Chronic Fatigue Syndrome* which struck me severely 12 years ago. One of the problems with CFS victims, as I am sure you know, is that we have problems absorbing and/or using minerals. As a result we often have insomnia, heart palpitations and multitudes of intestinal problems.

A friend told me about coral calcium. She sent me a tape by Dr. Robert Barefoot. I was skeptical because someone else had sent me coral calcium that came in little tea bags and I had tried it with no noticeable benefit. But I value this friends nutritional advise and out of honor for our friendship I listened to the tape. It was so educational. It opened up, for me, a whole new understanding of the need for calcium in the body. I loved the information and determined to try some.

I got my first bottle and opened a cap and dumped it in my mouth since I seem to absorb better when I do that and within two minutes I felt the most amazing things in my body. Peace would be the best word to describe it. And from that day on I never have had the stress in my chest I had, had for 12 years prior. And my digestion is wonderful now; no acid reflux anymore. And I have NO heart palpitations at all.

This product is more wonderful to me than I can say. Unless you have had constant heart stress and other calcium/magnesium related problems long term, you cannot imagine how wonderful it is to go through a day without those problems. It is like getting out of prison.

I have all my friends and family on this stuff and they ALL love it for various reasons. That is the beauty of getting your mineral needs met. Your body will use them to do the unique repairs that you need. The body is so smart. If you give it the tools to work with it will literally work wonders for you.

Thank you for a product that has been like a miracle for me.
Donna Crow
813 SE Crescent Place
Newport, Or 97465
541-574-1947

#4. Hi to everyone,
Just wanted to let you all know that I've been using the Coral Calcium, and it is definitely helping me. I am especially excited over the fact that I am sleeping better. My usual night activity is *frequent urination*, getting up 6 to 8 times in a 8 hour period to use the bathroom, plus I wake up in pain all through the night. Since the very 1st. night, I slept at least 4 hours straight before I had to relieve my bladder, then I took another calcium (not sure if it was necessary at that point) and slept like a baby another 4 hours. It's wonderful. This happens every night now. I have had such a sleep deficit for so long. Now some more good news: I have less pain. Oh Thank God ! I have *Fibromyalgia*, and after years of disability due to such horrible, constant pain, a wheel chair, and a walker, I have hope of getting better, and I'm not so fatigued. To have any less pain is a miracle, and such a Blessing. Now if I can start exercising and lose weight I will be so forever grateful to this product, and to Donna. Exercising makes Fibromyalgia worse, plus I have a back problem, a foot problem, and very weak legs. But somehow I know I'm going to keep getting better. THANKS to Donna for sharing this info. with me. I encourage you all to try it

also. I've taken other calcium product, but never achieved these good results.

Bless you all,   Joanie O.

#5   My name is Allen Jensen and I have battled *high blood pressure* for a years and have been diagnosed with diabetes for three years. Medication has helped me more or less keep both "in check", but has done nothing to lower either the blood pressure or my blood sugar level. Then, in October 1997, I was diagnosed with Guillaine-Barre Syndrome, a neurological disorder in which the nerves are destroyed by a :glitch" in the body's immune system. I lost a great deal of strength and dexterity in my hands, arms and legs. My active lifestyle of riding horses and a 30 year career as a telephone installer/repair technician ended with no choice but to take early disability retirement. In Mid May , 2000, I began taking coral calcium. Blood work showed a drastic improvement from tests in November 1999. My triglycerides improved from 1074 to 510, cholesterol from 380 to 210, and my blood sugar from 284 to 168. My doctor told me to "Keep doing whatever you're doing." With daily use of the coral calcium I am confident that I will eventually be able to discontinue all of my medications. Coral calcium has virtually given me back the life I was beginning to believe I would not be able to enjoy again.

Allen Jenson, Breckenridge, Texas.

#6.   With nothing to loose, we started giving our *crippled arthritic dog*, Bandit, 2 coral calcium capsules every day, figuring that if an average person takes 2/day to fight serious illness, then

Bandit, at about 43 pounds< should take 2. She takes her capsules in peanut butter ! That was July 1, 2000. Within just a day or two, she was eating again and walking out into the backyard and "using the facilities". Within a week she was walking normally. In 2 weeks she would actually "trot" out to the back yard, get on and off the couch, and come upstairs. By the end of 3 weeks she was actually playing "wrestling" with our 4 year old dog, something she had not done in 2 years. Our veterinarian saw her and asked what we had done to create the "miracle". He bought some coral and said that he would be experimenting on some of his patients. By August, Bandit was like a new dog. She'll actually run now !

Bob Zacher, Memphis, Tennesee

#7 My name is Lisa Macintire and my *18 year old cat*. "Tootsie", 9 pounds started *limping* about 2 ½ years ago and became very stiff-legged. She couldn't jump on things like the washer where she eats. She obviously had arthritis and was getting worse. About 2 months ago I started giving her 2 capsules of coral calcium every day, and in less than 2 weeks, she stopped limping. I kept giving her 1 capsule each day after that. In less than a month she started jumping and climbing all over the furniture. A check-up by the Vet showed her blood work, urine, etc. revealed no ill effects. The Vet's words were, "She's in perfect shape". The only side effect Tootsie suffered was "feeling GREAT". This coral calcium is truly a miracle.

Lisa Macintire, Memphis, Tennessee

#8.   I was diagnosed with **Multiple Sclerosis** inn 1978, and along with the disease came excruciating pain. In 1986 a pump was surgically installed in my abdomen, which put morphine into my spinal fluid 24 hour a day, and brought me modest relief. Last year, after 9 times in the hospital and 8 surgeries someone introduced me to colloidal minerals, which began to turn my life around. When I heard about **Coral Calcium** I thought, *"How is a calcium product going to help me ?"* Well, I tried it June 24th, and it didn't take me long to realize that this was not the run of the mill calcium. About the first of July, I realized that I had no pain. For the first time in 19 years I had no pain and I could work 12 hours a day without stopping to lie down.

Earl Bailley, PhD, Doctor of Divinity, Ohio.

#9.   Hi, my name is Dorothy Boyer and I will be 80 years old in June 2001. I have had problems at night time with my legs. They get nervous feeling and I have to get up and stomp around the room to get it to stop and then retire again. It is quite tiring to have to do this every night. My daughter has tried to help me with many kinds of calcium and magnesium products, some quite expensive and none gave relief. Then she found Dr. Robert Barefoot's coral calcium and said, "Try this." And the very first night I slept through the night without any leg problems. That was several months ago and I haven't had any night time leg problems since starting the coral calcium.

Also I am very happy because I feel like I can think again. I have been very active mentally all my life and just in the last year I started to have trouble concentrating and staying focused. After just a few days on this coral calcium I felt like I could think again. I am very happy about that.

The biggest thing though is that I have a congestive enlarged heart and it doesn't take much for me to get a really rapid heart beat. Just putting on a blouse in the morning would cause my heart to race and I would have to sit on the side of the bed and just calmly breath until it passed. From the first day I took coral calcium I have not had that again and that is the thing I am most happy about. It was very scary and it is nice to not be afraid everyday.

Sincerely
Dorothy Boyer, Newport, Oregon

#10. Your book did wonders for me. I had reached the point that *joint pain* was a part of my everyday life. Then, six weeks on coral calcium and I had become virtually pain free. Now, one year later, I feel better than I have in eight or nine years. Now my only problem is making my family and friends believe that being healthy can be so easy.

Rick Whedbee, Covington, Georgia.

#11. My husband Mark had *painful heel spurs.* He was advised to have surgery. He began taking coral calcium, 6 per day, and within 2 months he almost was pain-free. Within 3 months, all of the pain was gone and the doctors have advised that he no longer needs surgery. Coral was a miracle as Mark's job has him working on his feet all day long.

Betty Gosda, Illinois

#12.   My name is Patty and my husband was recently diagnosed with *prostate cancer*. My husband is 69 years old, 6'6", and works 12 to 14 hours every day from 5am to 5pm and later. Rather than expose himself to the horror of conventional treatment, he began taking coral calcium. After 3 weeks he had more x-rays and no cancer was found. 3 weeks later, hr went for a second opinion and had more extensive x-rays and once again, no cancer was found. God bless coral calcium.

Patty, Ponca City, Oklahoma.

#13.   First of all, I want to start off by telling you about my brother. Mr. Barefoot, you have spoken with my father several times about him. He has *lung cancer*. When it was detected, he had four lesions on his lung, one was the size of a peach seed. My Dad convinced my brother to take coral calcium. After 6 weeks when they ran another scan, 3 of the lesions were immeasurable, the big one had shrunk 60%. AMAZING !!!

Jeff Townsend, Kentucky.

#14.   I just wanted to give you an update on my father-in-law, J.W. Mitchell. As you know he was diagnosed with *bone cancer and cancer in the blood*. About 10 days ago he began your coral calcium program. His body went through detoxing for a day to a day and a half. He stayed in bed with the flu-like symptoms you mentioned, but he is doing better now.   He went for a bone scan and blood work last Thursday and we received the results yesterday (this is about 9 to 10 days of your treatment) . They now say that "there is no cancer in the bones or in the blood". The Hospice workers are in awe as well. The doctors now tell him that he may have a pinched nerve. He's a fighter and even more so now that he received the news from doctors at the VA that there no more cancer in his bones. He is convinced that he is still alive as a direct result of your coral calcium program.

Peggy Mitchell, Batesville, AR

#15. Just want to take a moment to thank you for all your help. What coral calcium has done for me over a brief period, is nothing short of profound. I can't remember any time in the last 29 years that I wasn't *in substantial pain*... that is until now. I have tried every pain remedy the orthodox medical community has in their arsenal, including narcotics, steroids, and anti-inflammatories, just to name a few. Most of them did a great job of messing with my head, a feeling I literally hate, but did very little fort the pain. I know almost nothing about the science behind this majestic mineral, coral calcium, I only know that it works. I have more energy, more range of motion, and less pain than I ever thought possible ! I know that there was a time in my life that I was pain free, I just couldn't remember how it felt until now. There are no words I can think of to adequately explain how much better I feel or what it means to me. Thank you so very much !

Best Regards, Gary T Schilling.

#16. I heard about your program from a lady who attended your meeting in Twin Falls this summer. My husband has a *rare genetic disorder called Alpha I Antitripsin*, which is genetic emphysema that develops because the liver is not functioning properly, therefore, the lungs do not function properly either. He has been under a doctors care for 9 years. After leaning about your recommendations to help heal disease, my husband began taking the vitamins and the coral calcium and has been on the program for 7 weeks. He let go of his drugs and monthly prolastin infusion program. He is now very careful about what he eats. He feels better and better every day and has just let go of his inhaler. He has seen great improvement. I would love to speak to you and share this miracle unfolding before our very eyes. You are wonderful... thank you for your research and efforts.

Mary Wiggins

#17. I thank you for the confidence that you built for me. After being diagnosed with *melanoma* with no real hope for treatment if it were to reoccur, I felt devastated. My surgery was done at the Mayo Hospital in Rochester which is suppose to be "world renown for its advancements in medicine", but that can't mean advancements in reference to the treatment of cancer. !! I now feel a sense of security for which I thank you. In a world of chaos and pain due to surgery, I felt that I was "drowning" in a sense, and thank-you, thank-you, thank-you, from the bottom of my heart and the hearts of my precious family in Minnesota. I have given your information to anyone who has felt the perils of ill health and you are indeed held in high admiration for your work and devotion to healing mankind !! YES for CORAL CALCIUM !!!

Marcy in Minnesota.

#18. I can't believe how different I feel after taking coral calcium. I lived with *constant pain in my heel* for months. I cold not jog because I could just barely walk. After taking coral calcium for two months, the pain is gone.   I am back jogging. I would not have done this if had not been for you.

Thank you very much, Russ Tomin

#19.   When one has been active all their life, it is impossible to understand the pain one suffers when the body is ravished by *Rheumatoid Arthritis*.   Knowing that it was important to stay active, I enrolled in a fitness class.. One of the activities involved lifting weights (20 pounds) with my legs. Due to the weakened condition of my legs, I tore a vital part of my knee. This sent me to the doctor and to physical therapy. When the pain did not go away, the doctor realized that the Rheumatoid Arthritis had taken over. I had been diagnosed 37 years prior with lymph edema which had caused fluid buildup in my legs. There was no known cure. The fluid must constantly be pumped out of my legs. This caused further damage and I no longer could have the fluid pumped out. I was in exacerbated pain now.   Then I learned about coral calcium. Within two weeks I Began to notice an appreciable decline in the arthritic pain. Within three months I became pain-free and I am off my walker. Also the swelling had gone down in my mouth and I could use my dentures once again. Even my barber commented on how thick my hair had gotten. I am now "72 years young" after only 3 months on coral calcium. I can't wait to see what 3 years on coral calcium will accomplish. All I can say is, God bless all those who have made nutritional discoveries, especially coral calcium.

Willette Barbee, Plano, Texas.

#20.   The "Cancer Answer". The first week of march 2001, my step-father was diagnosed with *Leukemia*. They wanted to start chemo therapy right away. He asked for a 21 day delay so he could start a nutritional program with coral calcium In addition, Bob Barefoot recommended vitamin-D and other minerals. On April 3, 2001 he went back to the doctors to run further tests on his condition. The doctors were amazed and totally baffled. They told him for reasons unexplained he doesn't need chemo therapy and that everything checked out normal. Hey folks, I thought Bob Barefoot had a screw loose when he claimed "coral calcium" could cure cancer. Turns out, he was right !

Jane and Sharon Gerding, Baker, LA

#21. My name is Susan Hedrik, age 49. I worked in a furniture factory carrying, stretching and cutting large rolls of cloth until it almost destroyed my body. I've had *back surgery* and suffered from a *painful bone spur* on my right thumb which two doctors told me would have to be removed by surgery. I also suffer from *arthritis* in my left leg. I was introduced to coral calcium and began taking it on January 27, 2001, and after 4 weeks "MY BONE SPUR WAS GONE" !!! I now can walk without a limp from the arthritis and no longer have to begin my mornings with a heating pad on my neck. For me, coral calcium is a "MIRACLE" !!!

Susan Hedrick, IR from Lincolnton, NC.

#22. I have a 14 year and 6 month Dachshund named "Andrea" suffering from *arthritis in her hindquarters*. She couldn't walk without falling over. She was unable to jump on a bed or the couch, even with the help of a foot stool I purchased coral calcium for Andrea and after 5 days she was becoming more

173

active. After 8 days she was jumping on the couch, begging for treats and running and playing. Andrea not only returned to normal activity, she also lost six pounds. Coral calcium also helped her teeth. Since she only has half of her teeth, I used to break her dog biscuit in half so she could chew it. Now, she chomps it down whole. As for myself, I have chronic arthritis in my lower spine. After seeing what coral calcium did for Andrea, I began using coral calcium myself. After 4 days I no longer had to take my prescription drug "Relafen", which costs over $3.00 per pill (I was taking 2/day). I now am a firm believer in coral calcium as I have personally witnessed what it can do.

Jack Polhill from Lincolnton, NC

#23. I would like to confirm that the use of coral calcium has been beneficial to my health. My *knee replacements* are deferred and my golf swing has improved. I'll be 74 this summer and I trust this sophomoric feeling is not second childhood.

Eugene T. Hall, Calgary, Canada

#24. I am an osteopathic physician practicing osteopathic manipulation in the cranial field. in south central PA. I have a patient who has suffered from severe *fibromyalgia* for the past several years. Recently she started taking coral calcium. This patient has improved dramatically. She has more flexibility and motion in her muscles and joints than she has in several years and she is nearly pain-free on many days. She has been able to continue a multitude of other medication, including chronic pain pills. The information in your books and tapes corresponds well to the science, the practical, the safe, the reasonable. I thank you for the time you have expended educating us.

Marianne Herr-Paul, D.O.

25.　　　　My mother, who has been on coral calcium for the past two months, paid a visit to her doctor to have her *cholesterol* re-tested. Her cholesterol had dropped 204 points and the doctor was amazed ! She is now a believer in coral calcium. I thank God for you finding this product that is changing people's lives and giving their health back.

Cindy Metzger

#26.　　　　My cousin Shirley had been diagnosed in May with *breast cancer and colon cancer*. She was scheduled for a double mastectomy and was also going to have her colon removed. You advised her to take the coral calcium and other nutrients and by July the breast cancer was gone and the colon cancer had shrunk. (Note: The October 1, 1998 issue of *Annuls of Internal Medicine* printed a Harvard study of 89,000 womwn that found daily multivitamins reduced the risk of colon cancer by as much as 75%). Her doctors, needless to say, are absolutely amazed. I can't thank you enough for helping my cousin, Shirley, as she means everything to me.

Patti Hernandez, Oklahoma City, Oklahoma.

#27.　　　　I am 62 years old and have always enjoyed good health. In July 1997 I was diagnosed with *prostate cancer*. The diagnosis was confirmed with a biopsy and an ultrasound. Two of six biopsies were positive with cancer. My doctors strongly urged me to take hormones and have my prostate removed. I thought about it but looked for alternative remedies. For six months I boiled Chinese herbs and did Qui Gong exercises and thought that this kept the cancer in abeyance. But in the spring of 1998 a second biopsy turned out to be similar to the first. "As a result of reading **The Calcium Factor** I received excellent treatment and eventually cured myself of prostate cancer. A third biopsy in July 1998 showed only one positive but reduced active cancer. I continued to take coral calcium and other supplements. A fourth biopsy in January 1999 showed that where the tumors had been, there was now only benign prostatic tissue. I had beaten the cancer. As a result I would strongly recommend that anyone suffering from cancer or similar debilitating diseases, should study Barefoot's book **The Calcium Factor** and take responsibility for their own health. I have yet to find anyone who has written such well-reasoned and scientifically based material. I have been taking coral calcium for 3 years and it has saved my life.

David G McLean, Chairman of the Board, Canadian National Railways."

#28.   In October 1996 I was diagnosed with *prostate cancer.* The diagnosis was confirmed by biopsy. In October of that year I started following Robert Bare foot's coral calcium regime. In July 1997 I had another prostate biopsy in which no evidence of malignancy was found. The regime outlined in the book **The Calcium Factor** improves the immune system to where the body can heal itself, without intrusive measures like surgery, chemotherapy or radiation.

S. Ross Johnson, Retired President of Prudential Insurance Company of America.

#29 "I am a physician, President and Executive Medical Director of Health Insight, S..B.S. and Health Advocate Inc., in the State of Michigan. I have extensive credentials and honors that reach the White House and Heads of States in other countries. Mr. Robert Barefoot has worked over the past 20 years with many medical doctors and scientists across the United States and in other countries doing Ortho-molecular Research on various diseases. The information has been culminated in the book, **'The Calcium Factor'**, which has been used technically as Bibles of Nutrition. Many people I know have thanked Mr. Barefoot for *both saving their lives and returning them to good health*. Mr. Barefoot is an amazing and extraordinary man who is on a 'Great Mission' for all mankind. I thank God for Robert Barefoot and thank God for coral calcium.

Liska M. Cooper, M.D., Detroit, Michegan.

#30 "Mr. Barefoot has been, and continues to be, an advocate for health and natural healing through nutrition and knowledge. He has championed the cause of well over 440,000 American women and children who have been exposed to the *toxic effects of silicone implanted devices*. Mr. Barefoot, one of the rare silica chemists in the world, has delivered a message of hope to these suffering individuals, who didn't have any hope before, but are now arming themselves with the book **The Calcium Factor** and are spreading the word, especially about the miracle nutrient, coral calcium. His work with hundreds of scientists and medical doctors, researching diet, has elevated him to one of the top speakers on nutrition in the nation.

Jill M. Wood, President Idaho Breast Implant Information Group, Boise Idaho.

#31   I graduated from Harvard University in 1942 (BSc Chemistry) and worked as a Research Director and in corporate management, and have been awarded two patents. Mr. Barefoot has been highly influential in my survival of *prostate cancer*, with which I was diagnosed in the fall of 1991. Because of his detailed knowledge of biochemistry, he has much more penetrating knowledge of the relationship between disease and nutrition, a knowledge not available to many trained dieticians because of their lack of biochemical background. With his expertise, he has aided me in not only arresting the progression of my disease, cancer, through diet and nutrition with coral calcium, but also reversing it.

Philip Sharples, President Sharples Industries Inc. Tubac, Arizona.

#32.   I am a chemist and have been involved in product development, specifically nutritional supplements. I have written numerous articles and lectured throughout the United States on these products, especially coral calcium, and the benefits of utilizing alternative medicine and alternative medical products within the U.S. healthcare regimen. Over the past three years I have traveled and lectured with Mr. Barefoot on numerous occasions all over the United States. He is recognized as a world class expert on calcium, especially coral calcium, and its nutritional benefits for the human body. I have personally seen Mr. Barefoot's information help a lot of people.

Alex Nobles, Executive Vice President, Benchmark USA Inc., Salt Lake.

#33.   One year ago my son Tim had *major back surgery*. Several disks had been crushed and three surgeries were performed. Four disks were removed , part of his hip bone was removed and ground to mix with a fusing material, then four cadaver knee cap bones were put into areas where the disks were removed. He has two titanium rods, two cross braces and eight screws in his spine. He started on coral calcium the day after the surgery. The first follow-up doctor's appointment showed that the fusion was doing great, exceeding the doctor's expectations. He said that this surgery was one of the toughest cases he has had. He said that he was amazed with the results, and told us to keep doing what we were doing. When Tim ran out of coral calcium for 3 or 4 days, he complained of severe back pain, which disappeared as soon as he went back on the coral calcium.

Billyr J. Stein, Ponca City, Oklahoma

#34.   The meeting that I had with you changed my life and how I think about my health. I am the person who's cousin's wife you helped. She took your coral calcium and minerals and she no longer has a *brain tumor*. My cousin's name is Gary Elias and his wife's name is Diane Elias. They live in Woodbury Connecticut and they are both grateful because Diane's brain tumor pretty much dissolved and has not returned.

David Querim, Connecticut

#35.   In November 1999 I was diagnosed with *prostate cancer*. My PSA was 244 !!!   On the way home, I listened to your audio tape. Talk about having the hand of God in your life !!! I knew in my heart that this is what I should do.. Once I started, I never deviated from the plan. The results were amazing after only one month !!! My PSA had dropped to 25.5. By May my PSA was 4.6 and I had my doctor and specialists scratching their heads over my instant recovery. My doctor said that he never expected me to live past the end of January, 2000. We also prayed and my doctor told me that "maybe the prayer worked" but it could not have been the calcium and supplements. Fortunately others have listened. My brother-in-law no longer has *high blood pressure*, ulcers, or indigestion. His sister-in-law no longer gets *cramps in her legs* and her *arthritis* is getting better. Her 5 year old grandson, who suffered so much from *leg cramps* no longer has pain or cramping and he can sleep all night long. These are just a few stories.

Bob Heinrich, Keremeos, British Columbia.

CHAPTER NINETEEN

SUMMARY

In this publication, an attempt has been made to demonstrate the importance of *The Calcium Factor* to both the quality and length of life. Of course, this is of increasing concern the older we get, because the older we get, the more calcium we need for our calcium-depleting bodies. Calcium, because of its *"king of the Bioelements"* function, appears to be the magic elixir for a long and healthy life. It is not surprising then to find it also playing a pivotal role in firing the first shot beginning life.

The following quote from the **The Role of Calcium in the Biological System** (page 149, 1985, CRC Press Inc.) shows that calcium is the trigger of life: "The unfertilized egg is poised only two minutes from the initiation of DNA synthesis. First, capacitation of the cell (rendering it capable) leads to changes in ion permeability causing *a calcium influx*. Upon fertilization, two ion fluxes occur in the short pre-replicative phase which are obligatory for the subsequent initiation of DNA synthesis. The first is an *internal surge of calcium ions*, and the second, an influx of hydrogen ions *resulting in the alkalization of the egg cytoplasm.*" There can be little doubt that the day will come when the calcium, responsible for firing the first shot in life, will be proven to also fire the last shot in life.

From the quotes and references previously given, the avid reader with a thirst for more knowledge can readily build a library of literature on calcium in the body. For the average reader who just wants to be informed about something of consequence to his health, he can feel assured by the sheer number of emphatic statements quoted from these men of science, that *calcium is the crucial factor in good health*. For example, another quote is, "The past five years has seen an *explosion of knowledge* concerning the properties and functions of calcium ion channels," by J. C. Venter and D. Tiggle, from the book **Structure and Physiology of the Slow Inward Calcium Channel**, 1987, Alan R. Liss, Inc. And lastly, physicians can be assured that the peaked health consciousness of the public today along with the computerized capability for communications will not allow the establishment to keep them from using this information to help their patients.

Another reason the medical profession should want to read, interpret and adopt this important information is the fact that *the vitamins and minerals are both so inexpensive and available*, and that the *pH test* is also so *inexpensive and simple*. Unfortunately for the physicians, the general public can readily attend to their own health. In addition, the pH test is so graphic that it leaves little doubt to both the sick and the healthy as to the long term state of their health. After reading the references from all the men of science about the importance of calcium, and then realizing that *the pH test is indirectly a calcium test*, everyone will, as the little boy said, "*want to be blue*" (pH of 7.5), just like their "*healthy friends*." Also, men of medicine should put their own economic fears aside and leap at the chance to beat cancer, heart disease and all of the other debilitating diseases of man, and go down in history as doing it in their lifetime.

For the scientific mind, a plausible hypothesis was given: *pH-regulated serum controls pH-regulated DNA synthesis and cell growth*. Also, the universality of these pH mechanisms in treating a variety of diseases and slowing the aging process was explained. The process of cell deterioration, whether by nutrient starvation or carcinogen stimulation with or without the onset of cancer, is in fact, the *"process of aging."* Minimizing and reducing these processes may be characterized as approaching the *"fountain of youth."* Using *the calcium factor*, we will be able to turn back the biological clock of life, a notch or two at least.

Not only will using *the calcium factor* help us dramatically improve the quality of life, but it will also result in a *dramatic drop in the burgeoning costs of medical treatment*. The two big killers, heart disease that strikes one out of every two people, and cancer that strikes one out of every three people, could be eradicated, and put in the same category as polio and diphtheria, being extremely rare. The now popular surgical gall bladder removal could become a rare occurrence. It is interesting to note that although Western medicine considers the gall bladder to serve no useful function, Mother Nature uses it to store the alkaline bile, pH 7.1 to pH 8.6, from the pancreas and liver. If too much of this bile is consumed by the blood (due to mineral deficiency), the gall bile becomes less alkaline (or more acidic) resulting in the precipitation of painful gallstones. (**Your Health, Your Choice**, by Dr. M. Ted Mortter Jr., Fell Publishers Inc., 1990). Kidney stones, which are created in a similar way, due to mineral deficiency, could also become a rare occurrence. The crippling diseases of aging could be minimized. Up to *one third of all elderly men and women* will accidentally fracture a hip. *Over one-half* of the elderly who fracture a hip end up in a nursing home, and up to one-fifth can die as a result of the accident. The elderly are also very susceptible to fractures of the vertebrae (back bones) and wrists. *Osteoporosis*, which represents adaptive decalcification of the bones, *is the culprit*. The ignorant use of pain killers will only permit the culprit to survive, worsening the disease until fractures occur. This culprit, like the ones responsible for a host of other diseases, could be shot down with *the silver bullet, bio-logical calcium*.

In America, where competition prevails, Dr. Benjamin Rush, America's first Surgeon General and the only medical doctor to sign the Declaration of Independence, tried in vain in 1776 to have medical freedom enshrined in the Constitution. He feared that "the time will come when *orthodox medicine will organize into an undercover dictatorship*". His fears were well founded as, in 1839, the American Medical Association (AMA) was founded and immediately began to ostracize from its ranks, the then popular, and what the AMA referred to as the "enemy", homeo-pathic doctors. Even the orthodox doctors were barred from hospi-tals where homeopaths practiced. Fearing financial ruin, these hospitals relented, barring the homeopathic doctors from their facilities. This practice of shunning the competition would be strictly illegal today, that is in every field except medicine, where it has become common practice. Dr. Rush, who was also America's first Surgeon General, referred to this practice as "*un-American*". Even Hippocrates himself would find his license to practice medicine revoked for practicing nutritional therapy, such as treating cancer patients with garlic and onions. Ironically, the action would be carried out by doctors who proudly serve under his "*Hippocratic Oath*". And this would happen despite the fact that modern science has more than proved that Hippocrates' teachings that *"All food is medicine"* was correct. The December 2000 edition of the Readers Digest in an article entitled *"The Health Boosters"* stated that science has discovered that garlic, spinach, broccolis, citrus fruits, grapes and tomatoes are all medicinal. The Digest claimed that garlic contained a chemical called allicin that acts as an antibiotic and may curb some cancers, that spinach contains lutein and zeaxanthin which protects your eyes as you age and also dramatically reduces macular degeneration, that broccoli contains 3-carbinol that reduces the risk of cancer (New York city's Strang Cancer Prevention Center), that citrus fruits are excellent sources of vitamin-C, folate and fiber, all linked to reducing cancer and they also contain limonene which is know to fight tumors, that grapes contain phenolics which raises good 'HDL' cholesterol, that tomatoes contain lycopene which haas been proven to dramatically reduce cancer of the prostate, lung and stomach, as reported by the *Journal of the National Cancer Institute*. Hippocrates was right !

Nobel Prize winner for the discovery of vitamin-C, Albert Szenti-Gyorgyi, once noted that *"there is but one safe way to avoid mistakes, to do nothing, or at least avoid doing something new."* This approach also avoids persecution, as innovation of consequence in all fields of endeavor has historically been persecuted. The greater influence the innovation would have on the public, the more stringent the opposition by the powerful groups protecting the status quo. Those that persist know that despite the many failures and the powerful opposition, *it is better to try and fail, than to fail to try.*

Ignas Semmelweis died of insanity caused by watching so many die so needlessly, never knowing when the doctors would finally understand the importance to human health of the simple act of washing their hands.

Similarly, also stripped of his license and credibility as a physician, Carl Reich, although supported by the explosion of research by the scientific community, was forced to wait for doctors to finally understand the importance to human health of the simple concept of *the Calcium Factor*.

Fortunately change will definitely occur. However, we are being endangered by the *pending avalanche of legislation* which is being sponsored by the giant multinational drug companies. For example, in April 1996, Congress passed, and the President signed into law, the **Health Insurance Bill**. The bill contained a rider from the *World Health Organization Codex* program that seeks to *harmonize* the governing and manufacture of health and medical products according to the standards set by the United Nations. The rider quietly passed. The Codex Commission Committee (90% of the Codex delegates represent *multinational pharmaceutical corporations,* who are concerned about the potential encroachment of vitamins and minerals into their marketplace) has proposed the following guidelines for dietary supplements:

1. No dietary supplement can be sold for preventive use or therapeutic use .

2. No dietary supplement sold as food can exceed the potency levels set by the commission.

3. Codex regulations for dietary supplements would become binding.

4. All new dietary supplements would automatically be banned unless they go through the Codex approval process.

What this means is that, as of April 1997, the Food and Drug Administration has the authority to close down all health food stores and will require a medical doctor's prescription for vitamins, herbs and other supplements. Thus the doctors with *almost no nutritional education* will be forced to participate as the drug companies eliminate their only competition, nutritional health, thereby maintaining the current trend in America of *disease out of control*. The result will be *legislated disease*. In Norway, where similar legislation was passed, the result has been the closure of over half of the health food stores with the remaining in jeopardy. The average American, **62%** of whom have chosen alternative medicine (according to a recent televised CBS documentary), will soon wake up to find that their choice of nutritional products has been removed from the market. The war against disease will continue to be lost and the average American will suffer enormous physical and financial pain. This is *"America's wake up call"*.

Only medical freedom enshrined in the constitution can blast away all of the *mountain of ignorance and indifference*. Until this happens, legislation, similar to the Alberta Government's Bill 209 (see page x), should be drafted and passed into law in America. This would at least force the drug-sponsored AMA/FDA partnership to "demonstrate" that nutritional therapy has a safety risk that is *"unreasonably greater than the prevailing orthodox medical treatment"*. Of course, as history has constantly demonstrated , this is almost impossible to do when employing a *"scientific basis"* for the demonstration. For the sake of the health of America, the legislation should be *reversed*, forcing the drug companies to demonstrate that the safety risk for using their drugs is not unreasonably greater than the prevailing nutrient treatment. If this were to happen, over 90 % of the drugs currently sold by the pill mill would *be removed from the market.*

Unfortunately, modern medicine has found a way to criticize the nutrient industry. They compare herbal supplements, which are in effect drug supplements, with nutrient supplements, which in effect are food supplements and then with a massive propaganda campaign they try to convince Americans that both are the same. The "Dietary Supplement Health and Education Act" which was implemented in 1994, was written by Congress to protect the American public from the biased interest of the drug industry and to give the American public the right to choose alternative medicine. Although a handful of people "may have died from herbal supplements reacting with drugs, no one ever dies from vitamins and minerals taken in normal amounts, while hundreds of thousands of people are killed every year by drugs. This is verified by newspaper headline stories such as the following:
a) *"Prostate Cancer Slashed by Vitamin-E in Study"*, Arizona Repubic, March 18, 1998.
b) *"Calcium Takes Its place As a Superstar of Nutrients"*, New York Times, October 13, 1998 ("reaching 1200 milligrams of calcium a day, cancer cell growth in the colon became normal")

c) "Drug Errors Kill Outpatients at a Rising Rate", USA Today, Tim Friend.

d) "Drug Reactions Kill 100,000 Patients a Year", USA Today, April 15, 1998 (quoting a report from the American medical Association).

Unless drugs are considered to be food, herbal supplements cannot be considered to be dietary supplements. Herbs are best described as "drug supplements", which can interfere with other drugs. Because of the enormous financial success of dietary supplements, the drug industry would like to trick you into believing that herbs are dietary supplements. By combining herbs with food supplements, the drug industry is attempting to give food supplements a bad reputation. Stories appear in the press "suggesting" that herbal supplements may have caused the death of a particular individual, and then suggest that therefore all nutrient supplements are dangerous. These stories are always full of passion and pain. However, although these stories involve only a handful of people, there were more than 106,000 people who died last year, 1999, from adverse reaction to drugs, and 50,000 people who were killed last year with anesthetics, and 350,000 people who were killed last year by mistake with drugs. When comparing these half million people to the handful of herbal supplement stories, the campaign to degradate the supplement industry becomes trivial. Although it is true that the drug industry has numerous successes, it is also true that the nutrient industry has numerous successes. The difference is that the nutrient industry does not have to kill hundreds of thousands of people to accomplish these successes. If there is to be fairness in the Press, then there should be articles on "Bad Medicine in the Drug Industry". Also, instead of using passion to bypass truth, the media should talk about the half million victims that the drug industry kills every year. Also, fairness would demand that there be a few articles on the successes of the nutrient industry.

The common complaint that food supplements have not undergone the same scientific scrutiny that drugs have, is unfair for two reasons. First, both the FDA and the drug industry refuse to carry out tests on products that they cannot patent and therefore profit from. Since vitamins, minerals and herbs are all natural substances, they cannot be patented. If the nutrient industry were forced to carry out these expensive tests by themselves, prices would skyrocket. The FDA, which has been given both the mandate and the money to protect the public, instead chooses to protect the drug industry. The ultimate result would likely be the retirement of most drugs. Even with herbs, which are drug supplements, the FDA refuses to fulfill its mandate to protect the public. The second reason for the unfairness is the fact that no one has ever been killed by God's vitamins and minerals, unless given in such staggering large doses that the same amount of anything would result in death. If the FDA and drug industry had put as much money into testing food supplements as it has into its propaganda campaign to discredit the food supplement industry, then most supplements could have undergone the scientific scrutiny that the FDA claims is missing. However, had this been done, the green light for supplements that would have resulted, would also have convinced most Americans to switch from drugs. Meanwhile the FDA spends our money trying to convince Americans that God's nutrients *"may be toxic"*. This is both hypocritical and ludicrous.

This problem is further complicated with prescription drug abuse rivaling illicit drug abuse. "Since millions of prescription pills enter the illicit drug market every year, some see a double standard in drug enforcement because of grants of leniency towards doctors (75% of physicians convicted by the courts of prescription drug crime kept their license) and their rich clientele who abuse drugs", Dan Weckel, *"Prescription Fraud: Abusing the System"*, Los Angeles Times, August 18, 1996. To compound this further, of the 20 billion dollars that the government spends on its war on drugs, only 80 million dollars goes to the DEA to investigate prescription drug offenses. That's less than ½ of 1% of the budget, and this despite the fact that prescription drugs make up 44% of the illegal drug trade. Thus doctors prosper selling *"drugstore heroin"*, readily made available by the drug industry, while most of those caught get to keep their licenses. And through all of this, where are the supposed protectors of American health, the FDA/AMA coalition ? They are busy doing two things. First they are busy trying to tell the American public that God does not know what he is doing as His vitamins and minerals *"may be toxic"*. Second, they are busy trying to convince the American public that Congress made a mistake when it passed the "Dietary Supplement Health Education Act". Logically, it is quite obvious that the American public does not need protection from God and Congress, but it is equally obvious that the American public does need protection from the FDA/AMA cartel.

The public should understand that the nutrient industry is based on the concept that the body can heal itself if given the natural nutrients it needs. World famous scientists, such as Otto Warburg, M.D., who won two Nobel Prizes in medicine, espouse this concept Today in America, almost everyone has heard a story about a miraculous cure using nutrients. This has become a major threat to the lucrative multi-trillion dollar drug industry, which has responded by oiling up its propaganda machine. Biased articles by the media are simply blind luck for the drug industry, but also results in great harm to American health. However, regardless of reckless attacks, nutrition will emerge as the Medicine of the 21st Century.

"If the doctors of today do not become the nutritionists of tomorrow, then the nutritionists of today will become the doctors of tomorrow", Rockefeller Institute of Medical research, New York.

THE AFTERWORD

Biological calcium has become one of the hottest topics in health research for both biochemists and nutritionists. The food industry has responded by fortifying dozens of food products with calcium. The dairy industry extols the virtues of calcium at every opportunity. Calcium has always been known to be good for you, now they are saying it is *great for you!* But *why?*

The truth is that most experts know only that calcium *works to maintain human health*, but they can't explain *why*. **The Calcium Factor** gives scientifically defendable explanations of both *how* and *why* calcium is so crucial to human health, and explains how **a deficiency of calcium** in the body can be *linked to* a great many degenerative diseases including *cancer and heart disease*. The book also explains how calcium deficiency can be both easily tested and readily corrected thereby providing preventive medicine for the control of many dreaded diseases.

Calcium deficiency has been shown to correlate directly with *the acidity level of the body's fluids*, saliva being the easiest to measure, and takes only seconds to test by licking a penny's worth of pH paper. Healthy adults and children will test bright alkaline blue, while the terminally ill will test highly acidic yellow. Those developing diseases will test mildly acidic green. An adjustment in life-style accompanied by modest and inexpensive food supplements will be shown to quickly raise a person's saliva into the healthy alkaline blue range, thus answering the concern of one little boy who emphatically stated, *"I want to be blue just like all the other boys!"*

Thus good health is both simply and inexpensively attainable from the knowledge expounded in **The Calcium Factor**. The goal of good health for the masses will not be easy, as the *undercover dictatorship* referred to in 1776 by *Dr. Benjamin Rush,* Surgeon General and the only American doctor to sign the Declaration of Independence, is now well entrenched in the power structure and has a vested interest in continuing *to oppose* preventive medicine. Thus, the freedom *to choose* and the freedom *to practice* the medicine of your choice must be *put back into* the American Constitution. Dr. Benjamin Rush tried strenuously, but failed, to have *"medical freedom"* enshrined in the Constitution. He stated " *The constitution of this Republic should make special provisions for Medical Freedom. To restrict the art of healing to one class of men and deny equal privileges to others will constitute the Bastille of medical science. All such laws are un-American and despotic.*"

The self-appointed protectors of your personal health will continue to stomp out medical competition and medical progress in the name of medical quackery. The computerized press makes it difficult for them to continue to do so, but a constitutional amendment enshrining Dr. Benjamin Rush's *freedom of medicine* as an equal to *freedom of religion*, would make it impossible for anyone to ever again impede medical progress, with the consequence being *"good health for the masses."*

ADDENDUM

Toxicity is defined as "the ability of a substance to cause injury to living tissue once it reaches a susceptible site in or on the body". Based on this definition, almost all drugs are toxic. However, when a doctor tells a patient that something "*is toxic*", almost always, the patient believes that the doctor means that it can kill you. Unfortunately, the doctor's common referral to "too much" vitamins and minerals as toxic is more than often interpreted as meaning that they can be lethal. For example, most people have been told by their doctor that "too much vitamin-A and too much vitamin-D are toxic". It is unfortunate, both because the doctor never tells you that the drugs he prescribes are indeed toxic by true definition, and because the vitamins and minerals that he is referring to are scientifically non-toxic when taken in reasonable amounts. The question then becomes, "just what is a reasonable amount and what is too much ?". Nutritionists believe that the amounts that should be consumed are often 2 to 100 times the recommended daily allowance (RDA). Scientific testing has shown that such amounts are both safe and effective. However, when seeking justification for the rash toxic statements, modern medicine resorts to studies where the amounts consumed are tens of thousands of times the RDA. Of course this is unreasonable if logic were to prevail.

When one studies the massive scientific documentation on tests carried out by world recognized scientists, one has to almost conclude that there has been a *conspiracy* to maintain the myth that vitamins and minerals can be harmful to your health. To present this information in a form that the public could understand would take several books. However, a discussion is warranted because of the importance of vitamin-D in the prevention of disease and aging, and because of the fact that, except for health stores, it basically remains off of the shelves, and when found, it is only in tiny amounts too small to be effective. Examples of such studies will be given and comments will be included where warranted for clarification.

VITAMIN-D TOXICITY

After vitamin-D was removed from the market following the toxic effects that massive doses had on seven medical students, the public, who commonly took mega doses (millions of I.U.s) daily and claimed dramatic health benefits, demanded a fair study. One of the first and largest was done by the University of Chicago medical facility, and took nine years to complete.

1. --- *Further Studies on Intoxification With Vitamin-D* --- I.E. Streck, M.D., H. Deutsch, A.B., C.I. Reed, PhD., H.C. Struck, PhD., College of Medicine, University of Illinois, Chicago, **Annuals of Internal Medicine**, Volume 10, Number 7, **January 1937**. (9 year study on 64 dogs and 773 people).

" Early experience with *impure preparations of vitamin-D* has lead to *a great deal of* **misunderstanding** and fear of over-dosage on the part of those who have little acquaintance with the fundamental mechanisms involved. Suffice it to say that *most of the earlier work must be* disregarded. "

" With eight exceptions, all of the 43 dogs receiving more than 20,000 I. U. per day per kilogram of body weight died spontaneously. " (between 8 and 120 days and an average of over 26 days).   **Note:** this minimum dosage was equivalent to 14,545,000 I.U for a 160 pound man which is *over 36,000 times the current RDA*. The maximum dosage was 500,000 I.U per kg or over 36,000,000 I.U. for a 160 pound man which is *over 90,000 times the current RDA*.

" Among the 20 dogs receiving less than 20,000 units/kilogram (equivalent to 14, 545,000 I.U. for a 160 pound man), there was **no evidence of cell injury**, insignificant weight loss, very little evidence of toxic symptoms, and with the exception of two dogs that died from distemper, **all *were in good condition*.** "

" From these experiments it appears that dogs may recover from extreme stages of toxicity and that whatever tissue injury occurs may be repairable. "

There were **no deaths** among the 773 human subjects whose " doses routinely given ranged upward from 200,000 I.U. total daily dose for periods ranging from seven days to *five years*. "

" One of the authors took 3,000,000 I.U. total daily (**7,500 times** *the current RDA*) for 15 days *without any evidence of disturbance of any kind*. "

" Both human subjects and dogs generally **survive** the administration of 20,000 I.U. per kilogram (14, 545,000 I.U for a 160 pound man) per day *for indefinite periods* **without intoxification**. "

" *Intoxification for short periods* **does not result in any permanent injury** that can be recognized by the methods employed in this investigation. "

" In view of the extensive experience in administration of vitamin-D to human subjects with a relatively low incidence of toxicity, and the correlation of the results of animal experiments with the observations on human subjects, we believe that **the burden of proof now rests on those who maintain the undesirability of the use of this form *(high daily doses of vitamin-D)* of therapy.**"

Shortly after this massive study (which found large dosages of vitamin-D to be both *non-toxic* and *beneficial to health,* and which was ignored by the American Medical Association) was concluded, the drug companies responded by introducing a new class of *drugs,* such as Dalsol, Deltalin, and Drisdol. These

drugs were nothing more than vitamin-D (over 50,000 I.U) with a filler. These expensive drugs consisting of inexpensive vitamin-D were so effective that the deceived public were impressed with these *"new drugs".*

2. --- *Effect of Massive Doses of Vitamin-D on Calcium and Phosphorus Metabolism* --- Karl P. Klassen, M.D., George M. Curtis, M.D., *Archives of Internal Medicine,* Ohio State University College of Medicine, **1939.**

" An adequate intake of vitamin-D *is essential* for the optimal utilization of calcium and phosphorus in the normal metabolism of the human body. "

" During four three-day periods, vitamin-D was given beginning with a dose of 200,000 I.U. per day. This was increased by 200,000 I.U. during each of the two succeeding three day periods. During the last period, each patient received 1,000,000 I.U. per day **(2,500 times** *the current RDA).* **None** of the patients showed signs of toxicity. During the last three days there ensued an increase in appetite and the patients had less discomfort. There was neither loss of weight nor marked change in the clinical picture. The blood pressure remained normal."

This study found that giving over *500 times* to *2,500 times* the RDA of vitamin-D, was *not toxic.*

3. --- *A Preliminary Report on Activated Ergosterol* --- (*A form of High Dosage Vitamin-D in the Treatment of Chronic Arthritis),* G. Garfield Snyder, M.D., F.A.C.P., Willard H. Squires, M.D., F.A.C.P., *New York State Journal of Medicine,* **May 1, 1940,** pp 708-719.

" We started our (four year) experiment by giving only 50,000 I.U. a day. This dosage was gradually increased. Finally *we came to the conclusion that is was fairly* safe *to start a dose of 150,000 I. U. a day* **(375 times** *the RDA).* During the past two years we have increased our dosage from 100,000 I.U.to a general average of 300,000 I.U. **(750 times *the current RDA*)** In some instances we have gone as high as 500,000 and 600,000 I.U. In most cases this average dose of 300,000 I.U. was maintained throughout the entire period of treatment. "

"We are inclined to agree with Reed Struck and Streck that **the hazards *of toxicity in high dose vitamin-D therapy* have been greatly exaggerated.** "

" The question of relative degree of toxicity of the various vitamin-D preparations in the treatment of chronic arthritis assumes great importance in the final determination of the value of high-dosage vitamin-D. The **original technic** of irradiation of ergosterol, followed by extraction of vitamin-D by means of alcohol, **was not designed** to obtain a product intended **for massive doses.** With the **new Whittier method**, the ergosterol is brought to a boil and the vapor is subjected to the activating influence of an electric current. This vapor is subsequently conducted off and crystallized. The manufacturer *claims that ergosterol manufactured in this manner will prove* nontoxic *if used in massive doses for the treatment of arthritis.* "

" The results indicate that the administration of vitamin-D, prepared by the Whittier method, in the high dosage of this study benefited the great majority of these patients in varying degrees. In a relatively high percentage of cases, *the degree of clinical improvement has been* marked and sustained. "

" *No serious toxic manifestations were encountered.* "

Once again, a sustained study, four years, of consuming levels of vitamin-D up to *1,500 times* the RDA, was both *non-toxic and beneficial to health*, and that the hazards had been *greatly exaggerated*.

4. --- *Follow-up Study of Arthritic Patients Treated with Activated Vaporized Sterol* --- R. Garfield Snyder, M.D., F.A.C.P., Willard H. Squires, M.D., F.A.C.P., *New York State Journal of Medicine,* **December, 1941.**

" There is no consistent change in the Blood calcium. "

" Most of the cases showed an increase in weight. One of the early signs of activated vitamin-D administration is a **markedly improved** sense of well-being and a definite improvement in nutrition".

" We believe that *the use of high doses of activated vitamin-D is not associated with any more danger than is usually encountered with other accepted forms of therapy.* "

Once again, high doses of the activated vitamin-D were found to be *non-toxic*.

5. --- *Comparative Therapeutic Value and Toxicity of Various Types of Vitamin-D* --- Chapman Reynolds, M. D. , Louisiana State University School of Medicine, *The Journal Lancet,* Minneapolis, **October, 1942**, Vol LXII, No. 10, page 372.

" It may be concluded beyond little doubt that **massive doses**, quantities **exceeding by a thousand times** or more the minimal requirement (note this is not the current RDA of 400 I.U., but rather the minimum requirement of 10,000 I.U required to treat arthritis), of *irradiated ergosterol*, manufactured in Germany in the late 1920s and early 1930s, may result in considerable impairment of nutrition, loss of weight, pronounced hypercalcemia, and abnormal calcium deposits in certain tissues and organs. There are **contrasting expressions** from users of the **electrically stimulated ergosterol (Whittier process)**, which reported **favorable results with no toxic reactions** and the serum calcium not elevated above the normal. "

" A study of the administration of vitamin-D leads to the belief that contradictory findings indicate that various workers were using different types of preparations. It is strikingly evident that massive doses of irradiated ergosterol bring about the development of toxic effects without clinical improvement, while use of electrical-discharge activated heat-vaporized ergosterol (Whittier process) has consistently been followed by clinical improvement with frequent rehabilitation, and with negligible or **no toxic** manifestations even over prolonged periods of intensive treatment.

This study shows that the original toxic effects that resulted from taking thousands of times the minimal requirement (over 250,000 times the current RDA), were not caused by the vitamin-D, but were caused by the impurities of using the solvent extracted and irradiated procedure to produce the vitamin-D. It also concluded that the same amounts of the newer and cleaner form of vitamin-D produced by the Whittier process was both *non-toxic and beneficial to health*.

6. --- *The Therapeutic Value of Electrically Activated Vaporized Ergosterol* --- Cornelius H. Traeger, M.D. F.A.C.P., Willard H. Squires, M.D., F.A.C.P., Emmanuel Rudd, M.D., Arthritis Clinic Hospital for Special Surgery, New York City, *Industrial Medicine*, 14:3, **March 1945.**

" Electrically activated vaporized ergosterol treatment given once weekly in doses of 1,000,000 to 1,500,000 I.U (**3,750 times** *the current RDA*) proved beneficial in the majority of the patients treated. "

" **The safety** of electrically activated vaporized ergosterol (Whittier process) when administered orally **has been established** and its effectiveness as an anti-arthritic means of therapy has been repeatedly shown. The previous findings have been confirmed and extended. "

Once again, the *effectiveness and safety* of the vitamin-D produced by the Whittier process was proven.

7. --- *The treatment of Arthritis By Electrically Activated Vaporized Ergosterol*, --- G. Norris, M.D., *Rheumatism*, **July 1947**, pages 56-60.

" For vitamin-D produced by the electrically activated vaporized process it is widely claimed that **in massive dosage it is of great value in the treatment of arthritis**, and that **toxic effects are so rare or so temporary as to constitute no obstacle to its use.** In a series of 164 cases treated at Cook County Hospital the blood-calcium level was determined before vitamin-D therapy was started, and then at six-month intervals: **no persistent hypercalcemia developed.** "

199

" A clinical trial has been started with a series of 40 patients. After 6-12 months (50,000 to 300,000 I.U. per day), a survey gives the following results:

Reduction in pain joints.............................. 23 patients (58%)
Reduction in swelling & stiffness in joints.... 18 patients (45%)
General improvement (feeling splendid)...... 31 patients (78%)

Of evidence of toxicity, the only ones observed were gastric disturbances in 16 of the 40 patients which ranged from a feeling of "fullness" or " a lump" in the stomach through varying degrees of "feeling of sickness" with the bigger doses.

Once again, the *effectiveness and safety* of the vitamin-D produced by the Whittier process was proven. One wonders with all of this evidence, what do the negative studies say. Well, the next study is a perfect example of a flawed evaluation.

8. --- *Intoxification With Vitamin-D* --- John Eager Howard, M.D. and Richard J. Meyer, M.D., John Hopkins Hospital, Baltimore, *The Journal of Clinical Endocrinology,* Volume 8, Number 11, **November 1948.**

" The age of the 10 patients given the drug (vitamin-D) as a therapeutic measure against arthritis varied from 33 to 68 years. The highest daily dose was 600,000 I.U.; the lowest daily dose was 150,000 I.U.. (each patient received one of four different drugs, and one patient received a combination of two different drugs). Duration of therapy prior to the onset of toxic symptoms was highly variable, ranging from two months to eighteen months. One patient received a quart of milk daily and another had been given calcium phosphate wafers coincident with vitamin-D therapy. "

" Eight of the ten patients had severe gastro-intestinal symptoms, namely, anorexia, nausea and vomiting. Weakness, fatigue and lassitude were prominent complaints of all ten. All our patients were given *diets very low in calcium* on recognition of their condition: yet hypercalcemia was slow to regress. It seems likely that the bones were the major source of the excess calcium in the serum."

" Seven of the ten arthritic patients *insisted that their joint symptoms were improved* during the period of vitamin-D administration. The patients reported that *the discomfort in their joints had decreased* within two weeks after beginning to take the drug. After withdrawal of the drug, several patients complained of sharp increases in arthritic discomfort."

NOTE:

1. This study had *only 10 participants*, compared to the previous studies with up to hundreds of participants, to which *five different drugs* were given.

2. Five of the patients were given the *impure, alcohol-extracted ergosterol* which *had already been demonstrated* in numerous studies to cause *discomfort*, which was *reversible*. This, in effect, reduces the study down to only five significant patients who were taking different drugs.

3. *The removal of calcium from their diet* at the onset of toxic symptoms (headaches and stomach aches) probably resulted in a dramatic aggravation of the symptoms as their arthritis was *caused* by calcium deficiency in the first place, and, by the authors' own admissions, *"the bones were the major source of calcium in the serum"* and not the dietary calcium.

4. Two of the ten patients *(20%)* were taking calcium supplements (wafers and milk). Their symptoms were never separately identified. Were they in the "impure ergosterol" group ? With so many factors, including the fact that the five indivduals taking the pure vitamin-D were all on different drugs, and with so few participants, it is *impossible to draw any valid conclusions*.

5. Although the authors reported toxic effects, the patients *all insisted* that their arthritic conditions had *dramatically improved*.

6. In this study with so many variables on so few patients, *the results* have to be, at best, *inconclusive*, especially since they are in contradiction to the much larger studies where the variables were controlled.

9. --- *A Ten Year Report on the Use of Natural Food Diet With Vitamin-D* -- Roger T. Farley, M.D. and Herbert F. Spierling, M.D., *Medical Times*, **October 1948**.

" The diet in arthritis treatment is based on the concept of fundamental physiology of nutrition: natural raw food, *unprocessed*. In all cases of arthritis, the use of white flour in any form is prohibited, and there should be no scorched fats, no creamed foods, no well cooked meals, no breaded meats, no fried foods, and no refined sugar. Patients may have the following: all vegetables, all fruits, unroasted nuts and honey, all meats, all sea food, eggs, aged cheese, whole wheat or rye bread, and butter."

" In the management of arthritis, one of **the most dependable and powerful agents** on speeding the arrest and recovery **is vitamin-D**. We began treatment (100 patients) with a daily dosage of 50,000 I.U., increasing at 3 to 5 day periods 50,000 I.U. until indications of improvement became clear. In the hospital, under strict management and research, we have run from 50,000 to 500,000 I.U. daily for periods of three weeks. On reduction of dosage, the *kidneys seem to have* **suffered no permanent damage,** *the urine showing no casts, no blood. In this research there has been* **no showing of hyper-calcemia.** "

O nce again, the *effectiveness and safety* of the vitamin-D, using amounts *1,250 times* the RDA, produced by the Whittier process was proven

10. --- *Vitamin-D: Too Much of a Good Thing* --- K.A. Fackleman, *Science News*, **May 1992**.

"In the United States, milk has been fortified with vitamin-D since the 1930s, a policy that has greatly reduced (from 80% to practically 0%) the incidence of rickets."

" Ellen W. Seely and her colleagues identified 7 adults and a 15 month old girl with unexplained vitamin-D poisoning. Too much vitamin-D results in **undesirably high** concentrations of the mineral calcium in the blood which **can cause** fatigue, weight loss, and in severe cases, irreversible kidney and cardiovascular damage (no proof provided). The scientists traced the problem to milk produced by a local dairy. The Food and Drug Administration recommends that milk contain 400 I.U. of vitamin-D: however, at least one batch contained 232,565 I.U. per quart. Eleven additional cases of vitamin-D toxicity were not included in the study. However, **the vast majority *of people who drank the milk (tens of thousands)* showed no sign of ill health *caused by vitamin-D.***

NOTE: This is a typical scare tactic report which only " *suggests*" that vitamin-D "*can cause*" toxic symptoms (symptoms that are disputed as incorrect by the studies previously presented), and in this case did so (the amount consumed was *never discovered*) with 19 people, while causing *no effect* on *tens of thousands* of others. Also the toxic effects induced by the vitamin-D were never described. They were probably head aches and stomach aches that stopped right after the faulty milk products were removed.

11. --- *Production of 1 , 25-dihydroxy vitamin-D by Hematopoietic Cell* --- Helmut Reichel, H, Philipp Koeffler, and Anthony W. Norman, **Molecular and Cellular Regulation of Calcium and Phosphate Metabolism,** Alan R. Liss Inc, 1990, pages 81-97.

" Vitamin-D is synthesized in the epidermis (skin) under the influence of UV light. Alternatively, vitamin-D is provided by dietary sources. In order to become *biologically active,* vitamin-D must undergo metabolic transformation. First, vitamin-D is hydroxylated in the liver at carbon 25 to form 25-hydroxy vitamin-D, (25 (OH)D3). The next metabolic step occurs in the kidney at the 1 alpha position to yield 1, 25-dihydroxytvitamin-D, (1, 25(OH)2D3), which is the biologically active vitamin-D metabolite with *a potency that is* **100 to 1000 fold** *higher than its precursor.* Research by many investigators have established that 1, 25(OH)2d3 is an important hormonal regulator of calcium metabolism."

" The human **vitamin-D receptor, VDR,** is present in the classical **vitamin-D target intestine, bone and kidney** as well as in the parathyroid glands. VDR is also found in the melanoma cells, breast carcinoma cells and osteosarcoma cells where 1, 25(OH)2D3 **inhibits proliferation;** in the pancreas where 1, 25(OH)2D3 enhances the production of insulin; in the heart muscle where 1, 25(OH)2D3 enhances ventricular contractility; and in many other organs where it plays a **crucial biological role.**"

" In addition to the homeostatic function of vitamin-D, there is an increasing amount of evidence that vitamin-D has important effects on tissues and organs other than those concerned with calcium homeostases. "

" With regard to the intestinal epithelia system, the genomic effect of 1, 25(OH),D was shown several years ago when the *de vovo* synthesis of a specific vitamin-D induced calcium-binding protein (calbindin-D) was demonstrated. In our view this appears to be an essential factor in the well documented enhancement of calcium absorption by vitamin-D"

Although this study did not evaluate the potential toxicity of massive doses of vitamin-D, it did point out some crucial roles that vitamin-D plays in human health. Also, it introduced the **VDRs,** vitamin-D receptors, especially the VDR's in the stomach, which allow *consumed vitamin-D* with its attached mineral nutrient, to pass through the small intestine wall and therefore be absorbed by the body.

12. --- *The Effects of Light on the Human Body* --- Richard J. Wurtman, *Scientific American*, July 1975.

" The formation of vitamin-D3 or calciferol in the skin and subcutaneous tissues is the most important beneficial effect known to follow exposure to sunlight. Vitamin-D3 is formed when ultraviolet radiation is adsorbed by a precurser, 7-dehydrocholesterol. Vitamin-D2 can be found in milk and other foods and can cure rickets in children who are deficent in vitamin-D3. Investigators at the Washington University School of Medicine have concluded that **sunlight is vastly more important than food as a source of vitamin-D3**".

Although this study also did not evaluate the potential toxicity of massive doses of vitamin-D, it did point out that *sunlight* is *crucial* to the production of the more usable type of vitamin-D and therefore *sunlight is crucial to human health*. An example is *endocytosis*, which is the process that allows nutrients to be absorbed or "swallowed" by the small intestine which is covered with thousands of negatively charged, fingerlike pro-jections called *villi*. The positive end of vitamin-D is sucked between the negative villi fingers leaving the negative tail of the vitamin-D exposed at the surface where the positive calcium ion can attach itself, thereby neutralizing the charge. With no negative charge left to repel the negative villi, the villi now can wrap itself totally around the calcium-rich vitamin-D and draw the calcium deep into the base of the villi where it can be absorbed. Once this happens, the negative end of the vitamin-D becomes exposed and is repelled to the surface by the negatively charged villi, where it is free to entrap another calcium ion and repeat the process.

And finally, a 1997 study by the North California Cancer Center concluded that *"because the skin uses ultraviolet rays from the sun to make vitamin-D* (which has been linked to protection against breast cancer in other studies which confirmed that woman from states in the tier south of Kansas tend to get significantly less breast cancer), that the *risk of breast cancer is lowered by 40%, perhaps even more, by exposure to sunlight."*

Despite all this massive scientific evidence, the average doctor still believes the myth of vitamin-D toxicity. Recently, it was brought to my attention by medical pioneer, Carl Taylor, M.D., Edmonton, Canada that the medical community was constantly being bombarded with technical information *suggesting* that vitamin-D was toxic. Dr Taylor sent me an article entitled *"A Brief History of Vitamin-D Toxicity"*, Journal of Applied nutrition, Volume 49, Numbers 1& 2, 1997, James C. Moon, Ph.D., FACN, CNS.

Although I found the article a treasure trove of information, the article was basically "misinformation" as the only proof presented about the toxicity of vitamin-D was in reality *"toxicity by insinuation."* No where did the article provide proof or provide statements on vitamin-D toxicity such as *"concludes that ..."* Instead, referring to vitamin-D toxicity, it used words such as *"suggests that ..."*, *"may lead to ..."* and *"may result in*

..." . These words by themselves demonstrate the lack of proof in this article of the toxicity of vitamin-D. By using the phrase "excessive vitamin-D *may lead to hypercalcemia*", vitamin -D is then held responsible for the damage to health caused by hypercalcemia, when in fact, just the opposite is true. High serum calcium levels are a direct result of decalcification of the bones for the purpose of supplying calcium to the organs which are desperate for calcium. It is also due to a lack of sunshine, resulting in low calcium regulating calcitonin production and calcium storage inisotol triphosphate production. Calcium deficiency, due to lack of calcium in the diet, along with lack of exposure to sunshine, are responsible for hypercalcemia. Vitamin-D, produced by sunshine, allows the body to absorb large quantities of calcium and therefore helps to prevent hypercalcemia. Also, the sunshine that produces the vitamin-D also causes the pituitary gland to instruct the parathyroid gland to produce the hormone calcitonin, which prevents the decalcification of the bones. Thus vitamin-D *actually prevents the health problems that it is accused of causing*. The scientific studies that "suggested" otherwise did not include the other numerous health factors that play a major role in hypercalcemia. None of these studies meet the basic requirement of being *"multi year, phase 1, 2 and 3, double blind, and massive studies done on large numbers of individuals"*, that are requirements to scientifically determine toxicity.

Typical of articles attempting to perpetuate the myth that God's nutrient, vitamin-D, is toxic, the article not only provides misinformation, it also uses arguments that are not true. For example it states that "there have been no systematic studies to determine vitamin-D toxicity for humans". In the previous pages I have provided 12 such studies, *"all"* of which *"conclude that vitamin-D is not toxic."* Many of these were ten year studies done on hundreds of animals and humans. Studies that were carried out by our best scientists and doctors at our best scientific research establishments. For example, the Streck Report of 1937, *"Further*

Studies on Intoxification With Vitamin-D", which was done at the University of Chicago Medical Facility and took dozens of doctors and scientists nine years to complete, concluded that they found large doses of vitamin-D to be non toxic and, because of the correlation of their animal studies to their human studies, they concluded that *"the burden of proof rests with those who claim the undesirability of vitamin-D therapy"*. This study was followed up by other massive studies which all concluded the "non toxicity of vitamin-D".

Finally, this article did provide information that proved that vitamin-D, in the amounts such as 1200 IU and 2000 IU which they claimed were toxic, just simply could not possibly be toxic. It is simple because all one has to do is apply grade 8 math to the numbers provided in the article. The article refers to a paper *"Cholecalciferol Production"*, P.C. Beadle, where Beadle measured the vitamin-D production in the epidermis (skin) to be 163 IU per square centimeter in *light skin* per day and 69 IU per square centimeter in *dark skin* per day. The human body has about 20 square feet of skin or 18,600 square centimeters. This means that the human body can produce over *3,000,000 IU of non toxic vitamin-D per day*. Also, the article suggests that 30 minutes of sunshine per week produces enough vitamin-D for the human body. Assuming this to be true, and also assuming 12 hours of sunlight per day, the amount of vitamin-D produced in 30 minutes is 128,000 IU which calculates to "18,300 IU per day". This means that they are advising that "18,300 IU of vitamin-D are required by the human body per day" (which this author wholeheartedly supports), while saying, at the same time, that 1200 IU "may be toxic". Which is it, 18,000 or 1,200 ? The latter is ludicrous as the healthiest people in the world, the Hunzas in Pakistan, the Bamas in China, the Georgians in Russia, the Titi Cacas in Peru and the Okinawans in Japan, all of whom have virtually no diseases, all get about 7 hours of sunshine each day and therefore produce about 500,000 IU of Vitamin-D each day (their skin is dark). Thus the logic of the Ph.D.'s who apparently cannot calculate, lies in the ruins of grade eight math.

Other interesting studies have been done. *The Lancet*, Garland et al, February 9, 1985 issue reported that a long study had shown that men with the highest vitamin-D in the blood had 1.42% colon cancer whereas those with the lowest had 3.89 % (or 273% more cancer). *The Lancet*, Garland et al, November 18, 1989 issue reported a study of 25,000 in Maryland showed that there was 80% more colon cancers in the fifth of the population with the lowest vitamin-D in the blood. In a report from England, *The Lancet*, March 23, 1991 stated that 3 of 14 women who were treated with topical vitamin-D experienced a reduction of 50% in their malignant breast tumors. A report in *Cancer*, 70, 1992, pp2861-9, by C.C. Hanchette and G.G. Schartz entitled *"Geographic Patterns of Prostate Cancer mortality, Evidence for Protective Effect of Ultraviolet Radiation"* notes that areas in Northern latitudes, such as Iceland, Denmark and Sweden have far more prostate cancers than found in areas of more intense sunlight. A report from M. Frydenburg of the Urology Department in the Royal Melbourne Hospital in *Cancer Forum*, Vol.19, No 1, March 1995, pp 15-18, states that high vitamin-D in the blood may be protective for prostate cancer.

In conclusion, medical doctors are reading and believing the thesis that vitamin-D is toxic, and as a result, are *"perpetuating disease"*. Ironically, I know medical doctors who claim to have treated patients suffering from vitamin-D toxicity. This only proves to demonstrate the medical fact that *"at least 50% of all medical diagnoses are incorrect"*. The use of vitamin-D with calcium supplementation could make a major impact on the war against disease. All be to read **The Calcium Factor.**

Glossary of Names

INDEX

210

Importance, 41
Processes, 96
Regulatory Ion, 53
Research, 22, 30
Systems, 19, 69-71, 79, 127
Valving, 10
Workhorse, 53
Bladder, 82, 129
Blood, 6, 48, 53-55, 69, 73-78, 91, 95, 98, 107,
109, 124, 129, 150
Blood: Calcium, 145,173
Cell Counts, 105
Clotting, 17, 74
Coagulation, 20, 21, 26
Cholesterol, 77
Floe, 55
Low Density Lipid (LDL), 76
Letting, 6
Nutrients, 75
Platelets, 71
Plasma, 20, 26
Pressure, 75, 79, 83, 85, 108, 109,
139
Serum, 9, 54, 55, 63, 68, 69, 70,
77
Sugar, 124, 126
Vessels, 83
Body Electric, 103
Bones, 10, 17, 18, 23, 53-57, 70, 104, 108, 124,
130, 142, 143
Bowels, 43
Brain, 4, 30, 77-79, 104, 105, 109
Breathing, 17, 96
Bronchial, 17, 85
Buffer, 41, 50, 95, 96
Bursitis, 54
Butter, 46, 76, 77, 98, 108, 115, 117, 120, 122,
144
Buttermilk, 81, 84, 94

C

CAI (carboxyamide aminoimidazoles), 71
Calcitonin, 54
Calcium: Binding Protein, 10, 18, 19, 31
Chennel, 17, 59, 128
Deficency, 11, 13, 17, 19, 20, 28,
32, 55-58, 59, 65, 67,
70, 78, 80, 85, 86, 91,
92,93,95,97,102,133,
175, 183

Disorders, 59
Gulconate, 84
hydrogen phophate, 71
Hydroxide, 101
Ion Deficiency, 13
Lactate, 47,141
Malate, 47,141
Orthophophate, 54
Phosphate, 47, 52, 69, 142
Regulation, 22, 59
Rosette, 52
Signal, 16
Calx, 33
Cancer, 7, 19-22, 59-72, 74, 75, 80, 81, 90,
104, 97, 105, 108, 110, 112, 124, 126,
128, 129, 130, 133,144,146
Carbohydrates. 53
Carbon, 34-36, 48, 64, 105
Carbon Dioxide, 64, 105, 116, 145
Carboated drinks, 117
Carboxyamide Aminoimidszoles (CAI), 71
Carcinogen, 63, 129
Carrots, 46, 89
Cation, 37, 40, 43, 63
Caustic: Application, 61
Cancer Therapy, 68
Nutrition, 80
Range, 45
Serum, 56
Solution, 66
Cell: Biology, 19
Charge, 51
Deteriorization, 73, 80, 129
Division, 4, 17, 19, 32, 104
Fluid, 40, 49
Function, 10, 19, 73, 79, 92,
95, 96
Growth, 24, 49, 51, 95, 104,
125, 126, 129
Injury, 88, 146
Ion Cannel, 11
Ionization, 52
Membrane, 4, 28, 31, 38, 41,
50, 52, 53, 62, 63,
64, 65, 78
Mutation, 21
Nutrient Channel, 10, 68
Proliferation, 17, 21, 32
Spreading, 69
Surface, 37, 38, 40, 50, 63
Wall, 10, 17, 51, 111